THE FAMILY
HOME REMEDIES
COLLECTION

FIGHTING
DISEASE

THE FAMILY
HOME REMEDIES
COLLECTION

FIGHTING
DISEASE

Hundreds of strategies
for preventing, treating and curing
common illnesses and conditions

BY THE EDITORS OF
PREVENTION MAGAZINE HEALTH BOOKS

Rodale Press, Emmaus, Pennsylvania

Book Packager: Sandra J. Taylor
Cover and Book Designer: Eugenie Seidenberg Delaney

Library of Congress Cataloging-in-Publication Data

Fighting disease : hundreds of strategies for preventing, treating and curing
    common illnesses and conditions / by the editors of Prevention Magazine
    Health Books.
        p.   cm. — (The Family home remedies collection)
      Includes index.
      ISBN 0–87596–263–7 paperback
      1. Medicine, Popular. I. Prevention Magazine Health Books.
    II. Series.
    RC81.F415   1995
    610—dc20   94–24202
                                         CIP

Distributed in the book trade by St. Martin's Press

2 4 6 8 10 9 7 5 3 1   paperback

OUR MISSION

We publish books that empower people's lives.

RODALE 🏠 BOOKS

NOTICE

This book is intended as a reference volume only, not as a medical guide or manual for self-treatment. If you suspect that you have a medical problem, please seek competent medical care. The information here is designed to help you make informed choices about your health. It is not intended as a substitute for any treatment prescribed by your doctor.

CONTENTS

ALLERGIES 1

ANGINA 4

ANXIETY 7

ARTHRITIS 11

ASTHMA 16

CARPAL TUNNEL SYNDROME 19

CATARACTS 23

CHOLESTEROL CONTROL 25

CHRONIC FATIGUE SYNDROME 30

DEPRESSION 33

DIABETES 37

DIVERTICULOSIS 42

ECZEMA AND DERMATITIS 44

EMPHYSEMA 49

GALLSTONES 53

GASTRITIS 56

GLAUCOMA 59

GOUT 62

GUM PAIN 65

HAY FEVER 68

HEARING LOSS 71

HEART PALPITATIONS 73

HIGH BLOOD PRESSURE 77

INFLAMMATORY BOWEL DISEASE 81

INTERMITTENT CLAUDICATION 86

IRRITABLE BOWEL SYNDROME 89

PHLEBITIS 93

PNEUMONIA 96

PROSTATE PROBLEMS 99

PSORIASIS 102

RAYNAUD'S SYNDROME 106

SEASONAL AFFECTIVE DISORDER 111

SLEEP APNEA 114

TINNITUS 116

TRIGLYCERIDE CONTROL 119

ULCERS 123

INDEX 126

ALLERGIES

Can you imagine a world in which everything you thought was safe suddenly packed a potent, even dangerous, punch? For the approximately 40 million Americans who inhabit the world of allergies every day, the simplest things—trimming a tree, taking a walk or going out to dinner—can be rife with risks.

Fortunately, most allergies are mild. Hay fever, for example, the most common allergy of all, rarely causes anything worse than occasional sniffles, headaches or fatigue. But others aren't so harmless. If you're profoundly allergic to bees, for example, or to peanuts, seafood or antibiotics, a touch can be hazardous, even deadly.

INSECT ATTACKS

If you are allergic to insect venom, a circling bee, wasp or fire ant can be as dangerous as a stranger with a loaded gun. At least 50 people die every year from insect stings, according to the American Academy of Allergy and Immunology. A great many more deaths probably occur but aren't reported. What's worse, many of the victims may not have known they had an allergy until the message came, quite literally, out of the blue.

This doesn't necessarily mean you have to rush to the emergency room the first time you're stung, says J. Schwartz, M.D., a clinical professor of medicine at Case Western Reserve University in Cleveland. For most people, it's normal to have some pain, swelling and itching where the stinger goes in. "It's only an allergy when you have a reaction that's remote from the place of the sting," Dr. Schwartz says.

If you do suspect an allergy—for example, if you get widespread itching or hives or you feel hot and dizzy and have trouble breathing—get to a doctor immediately, Dr. Schwartz says. After that, you need to think about the future, because second and third stings tend to be a lot more serious than the first one. To forestall problems, Dr. Schwartz recommends the following steps.

Keep your shoes on. Bees, wasps, yellow jackets and hornets don't spend their days plotting to nail you. But if you step on one with your bare feet, its reaction is sure to be quite pointed.

Blend in. Like you, insects are attracted to cologne, aftershave lotion and bright colors, Dr. Schwartz says. When you go camping, don't advertise your presence. Eschew fancy fragrances and wear subdued colors, he suggests.

Put away the food. "As you may have noticed when you put out a picnic table, they come from miles," Dr. Schwartz says. To keep hungry insects away from your buffet, cover the food as soon as you're done eating. Mop up spilled soft drinks and cookie crumbs as well.

If you have to spend a lot of time outdoors, you probably should consider immunotherapy, Dr. Schwartz says. "The protection rate has been very high. People who have been restung after completing the treatments don't seem to have any more trouble."

Of course, not all offenders lurk outside. Sometimes the worst enemy can be found right at home, at the same table, even on your plate.

FOOD ALLERGIES

Matt lives a thousand miles from the ocean, but he loves seafood. Crab, lobster, octopus, mackerel—he loves it all. But not scallops. He never, ever eats scallops. "If I eat them, I throw up," he explains. "It happens every time. Even if I only eat one, I'll be in the bathroom all night. I used to like them, but now I don't even like to be in the same room with them."

Actually, food allergies like this are uncommon, probably bothering only two or three people out of a hundred. Scallops and other shellfish are often to blame, although foods as varied as eggs, corn, milk, white fish and peanuts also cause trouble. Some people break out in hives when they eat the wrong foods; others have headaches, diarrhea or nausea. Although it's rare, some people can die from eating the wrong foods.

As with hay fever, the best remedy—in fact, the only remedy—

for food allergies is to stay away from foods that make you sick, says Philip Norman, M.D., of Johns Hopkins University School of Medicine in Baltimore. Of course, your doctor will want to be sure you really are allergic to something—that scrumptious, succulent shrimp, for example—before ordering you to give it up for good. Skin tests, this time with isolated food allergens, can usually nail it down.

TRIAL BY ELIMINATION

Unfortunately, people with food allergies are usually allergic not to one food but to whole groups of foods—shellfish, dairy products and certain grains, for example. It can be tricky knowing which food or group of foods is to blame. To find out which foods are friends and which are foes, your doctor may want to put you on an elimination diet.

The first thing he'll ask you to do is to keep a food diary, in which you will list *everything* you eat. (Be specific: Don't write "salad" when you really ate lettuce, tomatoes and onions.) At the same time, you'll keep a careful record of any physical symptoms that may be related to your diet.

Once your doctor narrows the list to a few suspects, you'll start the elimination process. This means that you'll give up, one at a time, the foods that might be causing you trouble. Suppose, for example, you see from your diary that every day you drank milk, you also got a stomachache. For the next week, you'll leave milk alone. If you don't get a stomachache (or whatever other symptoms you've been having), then you may have found the problem.

Of course, you might be allergic to other foods as well, so you may have to repeat this process several times. The only "cure" is to avoid the foods you're allergic to. Occasionally, however, people do become less sensitive. After a few months—or a few years—you can invite the banished foods, a little bit at a time, back to your table to see if things have changed.

ANGINA

Nearly three million Americans have experienced an angina attack, which usually lasts about ten minutes. It's not the same as a heart attack, but because of its chest-crushing severity, it often seems like one. And failing to control angina makes you an ideal candidate for a heart attack. Angina is one of the first signs of serious heart disease.

If you've already been diagnosed with angina, your doctor probably has you on medication. But here are some home treatments that can help you manage or even reverse angina.

Eat vegetarian. A steak-and-potatoes diet (with extra butter and sour cream) may have caused your angina by boosting the levels of cholesterol in your blood, but a strict vegetarian diet may help cure it—often sooner than you may think. Dean Ornish, M.D., director of the Preventive Medicine Research Institute in Sausalito, California, and author of *Dr. Dean Ornish's Program for Reversing Heart Disease*, recommends that people make comprehensive changes in their diet and lifestyle. He suggests a low-fat vegetarian diet that includes *no* animal products except for skim milk, egg whites and nonfat yogurt.

"When they follow this diet, most people find that the severity and frequency of angina pain diminish markedly within a few weeks, or even a few days," says Dr. Ornish. A vegetarian diet can also prevent angina pain and help keep arteries clean, because dietary cholesterol is present only in meat, milk, egg yolks and other animal products. And those foods also are high in saturated fats, which your body converts to cholesterol.

If you eat meat, go lean and light. If you still want to eat meat, fish or poultry, you should limit it to no more than three to four ounces daily. Also, choose cuts that are lean and trimmed of all visible fat. If you eat ground beef, it should be labeled extra lean. Be sure to avoid cholesterol-rich organ meats such as liver, kidney and heart. And remove all skin from poultry before cooking.

Boost your vitamins—A, C and E. Here's another benefit of a low-fat vegetarian diet: It's rich in the antioxidant vitamins A, C and E—three nutrients that have been found to help prevent or control angina.

"If your diet consists mainly of vegetables, fruits and whole grains, then you're getting all the key nutrients you need," says Frank E. Rasler, M.D., an emergency room physician and a researcher at Emory University School of Public Health in Atlanta.

Take aspirin. Taking aspirin regularly, according to a dosage regimen recommended by your physician, can reduce heart attack risk. A dose as small as one baby aspirin daily has helped patients with unstable angina—the kind that can hit you when you're resting or even sleeping.

"It appears that aspirin helps prevent blood clots," says George Beller, M.D., professor of medicine and head of the Division of Cardiology at the University of Virginia School of Medicine in Charlottesville. If clots form too easily, your blood can't get through the narrowed artery, and that blockage could trigger a heart attack.

Caution: Be sure to get your doctor's approval before starting on aspirin. Even though it is an over-the-counter drug, aspirin can have side effects, and it could interact with other medications you may be taking.

Get a regular workout. Even though angina pain is sometimes triggered by exercise, you should still work out regularly. Exercise helps improve blood flow to the heart, and it also relieves the stress that helps trigger angina attacks.

"When patients start an exercise program, they may experience angina with increased exercise levels," says Dr. Beller.

The answer: Exercise until you begin to feel the onset of discomfort or pain, then stop until the pain subsides—which may require taking a nitroglycerin pill. Often you can then continue, and the pain will not return. Ultimately, an exercise regimen will improve exercise tolerance, with angina occurring only with greater exercise stress than when you first started.

Exercise good judgment. People with angina need to exercise certain precautions. For instance, inhaling carbon monoxide can trigger an angina attack, so if you run, do it *away* from traffic.

If you live in an urban environment, try to exercise indoors. In fact, just being exposed to everyday levels of carbon monoxide can cause angina prematurely in some people, says Sidney Gottlieb, M.D., a cardiologist and associate professor of medicine at Johns Hopkins Medical Institutions in Baltimore.

Also, exercising in the bitter cold can trigger angina attacks in some people. So for winter workouts, be sure to cover your face with a scarf.

Raise your headboard. If you experience angina attacks at night, raising the head of your bed three or four inches can reduce the number of attacks, says cardiologist R. Gregory Sachs, M.D., assistant professor of medicine at Columbia University College of Physicians and Surgeons in New York City. Sleeping in this position makes more blood pool in your legs, so not so much returns to the heart's narrowed arteries. And it may help reduce the need for nitroglycerin, the drug of choice for stopping angina pain. You should check with your doctor, however, before reducing any regular medication.

Put your foot down. If you do get angina attacks at night, Dr. Sachs suggests an alternative to reaching for a nitroglycerin tablet. Simply sit on the edge of the bed with your feet on the floor. "It is equivalent to the effect of nitroglycerin," he says. If you don't feel your symptoms begin to subside quickly, then reach for your medication.

ANXIETY

Do you feel like something horrible is about to happen, but you're not sure what? Do you feel apprehension and dread even when everything around you is peaceful and calm? Do you feel a knot in your gut at the thought of making a speech, catching an airplane or going to dinner with your spouse's boss? If so, you're suffering from an all-too-common condition known as anxiety.

Everyone feels some anxiety. To a certain degree it's natural— even good. But too much anxiety can crush you—mentally and physically. Some of the common symptoms of anxiety are clammy hands, dry mouth, trembling, rapid heartbeat or breathing, headaches and drug or alcohol abuse. Serious cases can bring nausea, vomiting or diarrhea.

For some people, anxiety comes at the drop of a hat, while others feel anxiety only at the drop of a bomb. "Each person has a threshold of sensitivity," says psychiatrist Alexander Bystritsky, M.D., director of the Anxiety Disorders Program at the University of California, Los Angeles. If your threshold is too low, if you're one who gets anxiety at the drop of a hat, you can learn to keep your head on. You can control anxiety.

When it comes to anxiety, you have many treatment options. There's no reason for you to live in fear anymore! The simplest treatments can even be done on your own.

Banish catastrophic thinking. Anxiety can transform ordinary life into a string of catastrophes. But the string can be cut by asking yourself some key questions, says Michelle Craske, Ph.D., assistant professor of psychology at the University of California, Los Angeles. Ask yourself: Am I inflating events and situations, making them into something they're not? Where's the real evidence of impending danger and doom?

Take this scenario: You're an accountant's wife worrying that he's in some danger at the office, so you call him 15 times a day— making him lose all track of his debits and credits. The calls threaten his career and your marriage; they obviously have to stop.

FRETTING OR PHOBIA?

Frank Hughes is terrified of dogs. The 84-year-old man is convinced that their sole purpose on this earth is to bite him. Large or small, black or white, Doberman or Chihuahua, it doesn't matter. Deep in the heart of every mutt is a secret determination to bite, tear, mutilate or otherwise hurt Frank.

If he sees a neighbor walking down the street with something attached to a leash, Frank will cross to the other side. If he visits a relative whose dog comes prancing up to the car, Frank will stay in the car until the dog is politely removed.

You could say Frank is afraid of dogs. But Michael Kozak, Ph.D., a psychologist at the Medical College of Pennsylvania's Center for the Treatment and Study of Anxiety, is more likely to say that Frank has a phobia.

Should you try to overcome a phobia? It depends on how severely it affects your life, says Dr. Kozak. "I've got a friend who's afraid of bats, for example, but she lives in an urban area. So the only way her phobia disrupts her life is that she won't go into the small animal house at the zoo." Her phobia doesn't disrupt her life in any big way, so she does nothing about it.

When the disruptions are significant, however, you might want to use a simple behavioral technique to get rid of them, suggests Dr. Kozak. The technique is called exposure. All you have to do is periodically expose yourself to whatever it is you're afraid of for an hour or two at a time.

Walking out into the middle of a bridge high over the water and standing there for a couple of hours might not sound like much. But to someone who's afraid of bridges, the thought alone is terrifying. "What I do is park my car and walk with the patient to the middle of the bridge," says Dr. Kozak. "We stand there for a while, then walk back and forth repeatedly." It generally doesn't take too many sessions to eliminate the phobia, he adds. But the total number of hours it does take will vary from person to person: there's no magic formula.

Ask yourself: What kind of danger could my husband possibly be in at the office? Has he ever been endangered there before? What are the real odds that he's in danger? If something did happen—say he got smothered in red tape—how bad could it be?

Tape your catastrophe. An excellent way to get a handle on your catastrophic thinking is to make a tape recording of it: Talk into the microphone about the scenario that worries you, all the terrible things you imagine could happen. Then play it back over and over again and discover how you're overworrying, turning the normal into a catastrophe. "When you listen to something repeatedly," Dr. Craske says, "you get used to it, the emotion lessens, and then you're much better able to analyze it rationally."

Learn a relaxation technique. Controlled breathing, progressive muscle relaxation and meditation can all help to alleviate anxiety. Controlled breathing works by taking a deep breath, holding it for a few seconds, then exhaling slowly. Try it three times when you're feeling anxiety, suggests Carol Lindemann, Ph.D., director of the Anxiety Disorders Center of the New York Psychological Center.

Progressive muscle relaxation is simply tensing, then relaxing, every muscle in your body, beginning with your head and neck and continuing on down to your feet—one at a time.

Meditation can be as simple as repeating in your head a "cue" word, like *peace* or *calm*, over and over (perhaps while you do controlled breathing). With practice, you should be able to relax within seconds merely by repeating your cue word to yourself.

Set a goal. Each day you should set a goal—no matter how small—and do your best to achieve it, says Meg McGarrah, former director of the Anxiety Disorders' Self-Help Group Network. Suppose that every time you need to drive, you start to perspire and shake. "One day you might just make yourself sit in the car in the garage," McGarrah says. "When you're comfortable enough with that—it doesn't mean you have lost all fear—back the car down the driveway. Next day, drive around the block.

Then to the store. Then on the freeway." Before you start, you may want to practice your muscle relaxation exercises. If it helps, take along a buddy.

Lose control. Most people with anxiety disorders have a control problem, Dr. Craske says. They're perfectionists, they can't delegate responsibility, they're afraid things won't work if they don't do it themselves.

"Well, you can't do everything yourself," Dr. Craske says. "Stop grasping for control. Learn how to say no to people. Set short-term and long-term goals to manage your time, and stick to those goals." Let the world take care of its own problems.

Work it out. When you're feeling anxious, take a fast walk, a jog or a bicycle ride. "Exercise is extremely helpful," Dr. Lindemann says. "Anxiety and panic increase your stress levels, and exercise works off the excess."

Listen to the calm. There are many relaxation audiotapes on the market, and "they're about the easiest and cheapest way to learn to relax," says Dr. Lindemann.

ARTHRITIS

Here's a disease that's so common that nearly one in seven Americans already has it—and a new case is diagnosed every 33 seconds. In fact, arthritis is *the* most widespread chronic disease in people over age 45, even when you consider the untold millions who never see a doctor about that blasted pain in their joints.

When you *do* see a doctor about that blasted pain, he will usually tell you what kind of arthritis you have. Although there are more than 100 different types, most of them fall into two broad categories.

Inflammatory arthritis (or rheumatoid arthritis) is best treated with anti-inflammatory drugs, though diet and lifestyle changes may help. Noninflammatory arthritis (or osteoarthritis) results when cartilage in joints deteriorates from injury or excessive use. Weight control, proper exercise and pain relievers are the key treatments here.

Although arthritis is potentially crippling, there are things you can do that may help control it. Here's what doctors recommend.

Eat your vegetables. Researchers at the University of Oslo in Norway discovered that people with rheumatoid arthritis who began a vegetarian diet saw dramatic improvements in their conditions within *one month* after cutting out meat, eggs, dairy products, sugar and foods with gluten, such as wheat bread.

"A vegetarian diet is good, because the goal for arthritis sufferers is to cut as much saturated fat from their diets as possible and replace it with more polyunsaturated fat," says Paul Caldron, D.O., a clinical rheumatologist and researcher at the Arthritis Center in Phoenix.

Try something fishy. One of the best sources of polyunsaturated fats is cold-water fish such as salmon, sardines and herring. "They are rich in omega-3 fatty acids, which have been shown to have some minor beneficial effect on reducing the inflammatory aspects of arthritis," says Dr. Caldron.

Get hot on hot pepper cream. Research shows you can ease the pain by rubbing the joint with an over-the-counter ointment called Zostrix, made from capsaicin—the stuff that puts the hot in hot peppers. "You need to apply it three or four times a day on the affected area for at least two weeks before you'll see any improvement. An initial burning sensation at the site is not unusual for the first few days of application, but this goes away with continued application," says Esther Lipstein-Kresch, M.D., an assistant professor of medicine at the Albert Einstein College of Medicine of Yeshiva University in the Bronx who has done research at Queens Hospital Center in Jamaica, New York, and who has studied the effectiveness of capsaicin cream. "I also advise washing your hands immediately after you apply it—or even wearing gloves when you apply it—because it can sting and you don't want to get it in your eyes." (Sorry, but *eating* hot peppers won't help relieve arthritis.)

Use a dehumidifier. If the humidity is kept constant in your house, it can help calm arthritis pain that's caused by weather changes, says Joseph Hollander, M.D., professor emeritus of medicine at the University of Pennsylvania Hospital in Philadelphia. When rain is on the way, the sudden increase in humidity and decrease in air pressure can affect blood flow to arthritic joints, which become increasingly stiff until the storm actually starts. If you close the windows and turn on a dehumidifier (or run the air-conditioning in summer) you may be able to eliminate this short-term but significant pain.

Stay active. "Probably the most important thing you can do for osteoarthritis is exercise as much as you're able to," says Halsted R. Holman, M.D., director and professor of medicine at the Stanford University Arthritis Center in Stanford, California. "You will find that the better your physical condition, the less arthritis pain you will have."

Dr. Caldron recommends low-impact aerobic exercises and, if tolerated, very light weight lifting with one- to two-pound dumbbells. "Build up the muscle and tissue surrounding the joint," he

THE CASE FOR COPPER

S ometimes longevity confers respect along with age. Artifacts that were rarely noticed in their day take on new meaning and value as they persist throughout time. Such is the case with the copper bracelet, which for decades has been worn for arthritis relief and remains popular today.

Studies have shown that some people with arthritis seem to have difficulty metabolizing copper from the food they eat, leading to increased pain. That observation led Helmar Dollwet, Ph.D., of the University of Akron to theorize that arthritis sufferers may need to get their copper from another source. "The dissolved copper from a [copper] bracelet bypasses the oral route by entering the body through the skin," he wrote in his book, *The Copper Bracelet and Arthritis*. Dr. Dollwet thought this might be the only way arthritics ever receive the copper their bodies need—copper that studies have shown can indeed relieve pain.

Physicians remain somewhat skeptical about bracelets but don't entirely dismiss them, either. "I see people wearing copper bracelets, and they're wearing them because it helps them," says Elson Haas, M.D. "I think copper may have a role. It's possible that a copper deficiency does increase joint inflammation, and it doesn't seem that supplementing copper in the diet has the same effect as wearing it."

Does that make Dr. Haas a believer? "I don't necessarily supply copper bracelets to people, but I don't discourage them from wearing one either."

suggests. "You can exercise on a floor mat, in a chair, on a stationary bicycle or in the water. The key is regularity, doing it no less than three times a week but preferably daily."

Work wonders with watercise. Ask a dozen doctors about the merits of any arthritis treatment and you'll get a dozen different opinions. But ask them about exercising in water and a strange thing happens—they all agree.

"Water exercises are excellent," says Art Mollen, D.O., an osteopathic physician and director of the Southwest Health Institute in Phoenix, Arizona, who echoes the sentiments of many physicians. "Your pain will be significantly reduced in the water, and you become much more flexible in water than you are in air. I can't say enough about water exercises!"

Learn your food "triggers." "Some people with rheumatoid arthritis seem to flare up after eating certain foods—especially alcohol, milk, tomatoes and certain nuts," says Dr. Caldron. "Although there's really no telling what your trigger might be, if you notice your condition worsens after eating a certain food, then listen to your body and avoid that food." The same goes for foods that improve arthritis, such as fish and fiber; try to eat them more regularly.

Take time to smell the roses. When you're tensed up, you hurt more. "Many people use relaxation as an effective way of diminishing arthritis pain," says Dr. Holman. "It really doesn't matter what you do—biofeedback, meditation, even listening to music—whatever helps *you* relax. The point is to practice a regular relaxation period and then also to use relaxation when pain is particularly severe."

Slim down. "Being overweight can enhance damage to joints by putting excess pressure on them, resulting in worsening osteoarthritis, so I advise losing any excess weight you're carrying," says Richard M. Pope, M.D., a leading arthritis researcher and chief of arthritis and connective tissue diseases at Northwestern University Medical School in Chicago. In fact, being overweight increases your risk of developing osteoarthritis, even if you don't have it now.

Try slow dancing. Dancing is a good way to combine weight loss, exercise and stress reduction. "Many of my patients participate in easy dance routines created as part of an overall education and activity program that shows them how to exercise while protecting their affected joints," adds Dr. Pope. "Easy, slow dancing is perfect for those with inflammatory arthritis or osteoarthritis, because it's low impact."

Reach for the "right" pain reliever. Not all pain relievers are the same—at least for those with arthritis. "People with inflammatory arthritis should get more relief from aspirin or ibuprofen, but may get more stomach irritation with these," says Dr. Caldron. For over-the-counter pain relief without stomach irritation, he recommends acetaminophen. Recommended doses of these drugs should not be exceeded, nor regular dosing continued for more than three weeks without consulting your physician.

Use ice and heat judiciously. Although both ice packs and heat packs can provide some relief, don't use either for more than ten minutes at a time, advises Dr. Caldron. Usually ice is used to prevent swelling but may also douse pain; heat in small doses may promote muscle relaxation and soothe pain.

ASTHMA

Asthma means twitchy airways," says allergist Peter Creticos, M.D., of the Johns Hopkins Center for Asthma and Allergic Disease in Baltimore. "Your bronchial airways suddenly contract, you feel a tightness in your chest, you become short of breath and you cough and wheeze."

"In the under-40 age group, probably 90 percent of asthma is triggered by an allergy," says William Ziering, M.D., a Fresno, California, allergist. Tree, weed and grass pollens, animal dander, dust mites and mold are the biggest allergic triggers for asthma. "After age 40, it's about 50 percent. The other 50 percent is triggered by some form of lung disorder such as emphysema."

But no matter what the cause, asthma needn't be a life sentence. You can get your chest problems under control. "Asthma is a reversible disease," says Dr. Ziering. And you don't have to go to the Sahara desert looking for a way to reverse your asthma; there's plenty you can do right at home.

Stay out of smoke-filled rooms. People with asthma shouldn't smoke, but a recent study done in Canada found that people around asthmatics shouldn't smoke either. "This is particularly important in the winter months, when houses are closed up," says Brenda Morrison, Ph.D., a researcher and associate professor at the University of British Columbia in Vancouver, who conducted a study on the effects of cigarette smoking on asthma. "If someone in the house smokes, it leads to a worsening of asthma, especially in children."

Avoid night noshing. Going to sleep on a full stomach might also feed your asthma. "Asthma can be caused by stomach reflux," says Dr. Creticos. Reflux occurs when stomach acid backs up into the esophagus.

"Stomach contents may leak out and actually regurgitate into your mouth and then drip down into your airways while you're lying down or sleeping," Dr. Creticos says. "Besides avoiding snacks, you could also take an antacid before bedtime to cut down

BEWARE OF ASPIRIN!

If you have asthma and suffer from sinusitis and nasal polyps, you should get your pain relief from acetaminophen, not from aspirin or other nonsteroidal anti-inflammatory drugs (NSAIDs) such as ibuprofen (Advil).

"Taking aspirin or NSAIDs could make your asthma worse or may even be life-threatening," warns allergist Peter S. Creticos, M.D., of the Johns Hopkins Center for Asthma and Allergic Disease in Baltimore. Acetaminophen products such as Tylenol, Aspirin-Free Arthritis Pain Formula and Panadol are considered safe, he says.

Also, if you have arthritis as well as asthma, Dr. Creticos recommends seeing your doctor before taking any of the usual medications to ease pain and inflammation. Ask the doctor to prescribe an anti-inflammatory medication that will help the symptoms without causing asthma problems.

on your stomach's acidity." Theophylline medications, which are sometimes prescribed to help control asthma, may actually aggravate your condition by increasing stomach reflux, according to Dr. Creticos. If you are taking this medication and are having reflux problems, be sure to check with your doctor, so the dosage level can be adjusted.

Prop up your bed (or yourself). Besides cutting out midnight snacks, other ways to prevent reflux-induced asthma include elevating the head of your bed by placing it on bricks or wood blocks. Or prop yourself up with pillows to prevent acids moving from your stomach to your esophagus, suggests H. James Wedner, M.D., chief of clinical allergy and immunology at Washington University School of Medicine in St. Louis.

Go the fish route. Since Eskimos get asthma about as often as they get heatstroke, some theorize that a fish-rich diet may help *prevent* asthma. Although tests aren't conclusive, Walter Pickett, Ph.D., senior research biochemist and group leader of the Medical Research Division at Lederle Laboratories in Pearl River, New York, says it is conceivable that eating sardines, herring, mackerel and other fish rich in omega-3 fatty acids at least once a week may help lessen asthma's impact.

Multiply your vitamins. Taking a good multivitamin/mineral supplement and eating plenty of fruits and vegetables may also help, since some nutrients have been found to lessen symptoms associated with asthma attacks. Reviewing data from more than 9,000 people, researchers found that those with reduced levels of vitamin C and zinc suffered more from wheezing and other bronchial problems. Good food sources of vitamin C include citrus fruits, broccoli and peppers. Oysters, beef and crab are among the foods highest in zinc.

Get relief from caffeine. Although coffee has been shown to contribute to some health problems, it may be more helpful than harmful for many people with asthma. Caffeine, it turns out, has nearly the same effect as theophylline.

"A couple of cups of strong, regular black coffee will have a beneficial effect on asthma," says allergist Allan Becker, M.D., an associate professor of medicine in the Section of Pediatric Allergy and Clinical Immunology at the University of Manitoba in Winnipeg, who tested the effects of caffeine on asthma. But don't use caffeine as a substitute for—or in combination with—your medication, he advises, because it is good only for emergency use. "In an emergency, when you don't have your medication around, two cups of strong, regular black coffee [sugar and milk slow absorption] can provide effective temporary relief until your regular medication is available," says Dr. Becker. Relief can also be provided—but the effect will be slower—with two cups of hot cocoa or eight ounces of milk chocolate candy.

CARPAL TUNNEL SYNDROME

Yes, the computer has certainly expanded our horizons and given us the ability to perform lightninglike calculations. But along with every computer comes a keyboard—and human fingers that hit the keys with the speed of raindrops in a thunderstorm.

Unfortunately, the human wrist wasn't made for this kind of frantic activity. Hands that carry out repetitive tasks at the computer keyboard (or anywhere else, for that matter) may begin sending up protests of pain. This wrist pain is the screaming ouch of a disorder called carpal tunnel syndrome.

Carpal tunnel syndrome is like a traffic jam in the wrist, resulting from too much crowding in too little space. Nestled among the bones and tendons of the wrist area lies a major median nerve that leads from the arm into the fingers. This is the nerve that "signals" some of the small muscles in the hand and also provides sensation to the thumb and first three fingers.

Crowded in next to that nerve, inside the "carpal tunnel," are several tendons. When the tendons are overworked, they become inflamed and swell, and the median nerve is literally crushed within the carpal tunnel.

As the tendons swell and the tunnel size shrinks, the median nerve gets crushed like a piece of soft spaghetti. No wonder it hurts!

Although often caused by the repetitive movements of keyboard operation or typing, hammering or other hand-intensive job chores, carpal tunnel syndrome can result from just about anything in which your hands are used frequently and for long periods. A good start toward stopping the pain is to eliminate the cause (if you know it). And here are some other approaches.

Stretch your hands. To keep pain at bay, start off each activity with a series of hand-stretching exercises. "Anything that extends the range of motion in your fingers and wrist will help," says Janna Jacobs, president of the American Physical Therapy Association's Section on Hand Rehabilitation. "Open and close your fingers, bend your wrists in both directions—do various things to exercise your hands for about 10 or 15 minutes before beginning the activity."

Watch out for bad vibes. Although electric tools do quick work, they're a bad influence on your wrist. "True, there may be less force placed on your wrist, but the vibrations of an electric knife or other power tools could require a tighter grip to steady them and lead to another disorder called hand-arm vibration syndrome," says occupational medicine specialist Thomas Hales, M.D., of the National Institute for Occupational Safety and Health in Denver. When buying tools like a power painter or chain saw, look for those with special "vibration control" mechanisms.

Fatten tool handles. Placing foam rubber over the handles of brooms, rakes and other tools—or simply wrapping handles in foam tape to fatten them—makes them easier to hold, decreasing or eliminating pain. "If handles are too small, they can press directly on the tendons and median nerve in the palm," says David Rempel, M.D., an ergonomist and expert in occupational medicine at the University of California, San Francisco. But don't make handles too big, either—that also hurts wrists.

Sharpen your knives. Simple household chores such as cutting meat or clipping hedges can cause big-time pain for those with carpal tunnel syndrome. "Keeping your tools sharp or well lubricated reduces the amount of pressure needed to use them," says Peter C. Amadio, M.D., associate professor of orthopedics at the Mayo Medical School in Rochester, Minnesota.

Write with a light touch. "Using pencils with soft lead or pens with easy-flow ink also helps a lot," says Dr. Amadio. "And the fatter and rounder the pen or pencil, the easier it is to use."

"B" aware of vitamin deficiencies. Why do some people who use their hands and fingers a great deal develop carpal tunnel

IT COULD BE ARTHRITIS

W rist and hand pain is not always the result of carpal tunnel syndrome and could actually be the sign of a more serious illness, cautions physical therapist Susan Isernhagen of Duluth, Minnesota. In fact, she says, "if you get a crackly or crunchy feeling in your wrist when you exercise it, that's not a sign of carpal tunnel syndrome; it may be a symptom of osteoarthritis." You should have it checked out by your doctor.

syndrome while others don't? Some studies suggest that it may be partly the result of a borderline B-vitamin deficiency, specifically vitamin B_6. Although excessive doses of vitamin B_6 supplements may cause nerve damage, a low dose is safe. "Studies suggest that 100 milligrams a day of vitamin B_6 can significantly reduce the debilitating and crippling symptoms of carpal tunnel syndrome," says Hans Fisher, Ph.D., professor of nutrition at Rutgers University in New Brunswick, New Jersey.

Wear a wrist splint to bed. All of our experts recommend wearing a wrist splint whenever possible and especially at night. Splints are available at most drugstores without a prescription. "Carpal tunnel pain is usually worse at night, when body fluids collect in wrists and other body parts," according to Steven Barrer, Jr., M.D., a clinical assistant professor of neurosurgery at the Medical College of Pennsylvania in Philadelphia who has written numerous articles on carpal tunnel syndrome. "In fact, loss of sleep due to the pain of carpal tunnel syndrome is probably the most bothersome symptom of the disease."

Another problem: Many people inadvertently curl their wrists while sleeping, putting pressure on the median nerve and causing pain. "A wrist splint immobilizes your wrist," says Jacobs. In fact, you should wear a wrist splint whenever you're not doing a "hands-on" activity. (Wearing one during such activities may reduce range of motion too much.)

Take frequent breaks from "hands-on" activity. "If your carpal tunnel syndrome is related to your job, taking a five-minute break from the offending chore every hour or so will make a big difference in your condition," suggests Dr. Barrer. "Even a few minutes' rest can often relieve the pain you feel. Of course, if possible, try to completely avoid the activity causing the trouble."

Pack on an ice pack. You may find that the pain lessens when you put an ice pack on your wrist, according to Dr. Barrer. "If you use an ice pack [a bag of frozen vegetables works fine], wrap it in a dish towel and hold it between your wrists for 10 or 15 minutes, then remove it for about the same amount of time, and repeat. This will prevent a freeze burn."

Or warm your wrists with a heating pad. Others find relief by holding a heating pad or warm compress between their wrists to relax muscles, adds Dr. Barrer. "The best thing to do is try both and see what works for you," he says. "For some, it's heat; for others, it's cold."

CATARACTS

A cataract is a painless clouding of the normally clear lens of the eye. Left untreated, it can cause blindness. But this clouding has a silver lining: Surgery can restore lost sight in most cases.

While many people over age 60 do have some clouding of the eye lens and therefore some degree of cataracts, there are ways to help prevent cataracts from forming or getting worse at any age. Here's how to help make sure your lenses stay clear.

Drink your orange juice. "Our research shows there's a lower risk of developing cataracts in people who consume a lot of vitamin C in their diets," says Allen Taylor, Ph.D., director of the Lens Nutrition and Aging Division of the U.S. Department of Agriculture Human Nutrition Research Center on Aging at Tufts University in Boston. "We're still trying to find out exactly how much is needed for protection against cataracts, but we know it's at least two times the Recommended Dietary Allowance," he says. That amounts to 1 cup of orange juice, 2 oranges or 1½ cups of strawberries.

Get your beta-carotene and vitamin E. "Vitamin E and beta-carotene also seem to offer some protection," adds Dr. Taylor. He recommends yellow and orange vegetables such as carrots, squash and sweet potatoes as excellent sources of beta-carotene. Foods high in vitamin E include almonds, fortified cereals, peanut butter and sunflower seeds.

Wear sunglasses or a hat. "The most credible evidence shows that the best way to prevent cataracts is to protect your eyes from the sun's ultraviolet rays," says Merrill M. Knopf, M.D., an ophthalmologist in Long Beach, California, and an officer of the California Association of Ophthalmology. "Be sure to wear sunglasses or a hat when you're outdoors. And there's no need to spend $100 or more for a pair of designer sunglasses, since all sunglasses sold in the United States offer UV protection. Putting a sticker on them to say that is simply a way to drive up the price. The kind sold at your drugstore will do as well as those sold by your eye doctor."

Look away when the microwave's in use. Even small doses of radiation make you more prone to developing cataracts, so limiting exposure to radiation sources—such as microwave ovens and x-ray machines—is recommended. "I know that all manufacturers say their ovens are safe, and maybe they are, but I make a point of turning my head away from my microwave oven and closing my eyes while it's in use," says Dr. Knopf. "I do the same when I'm at my dentist's office getting x-rays."

Control your vices. Occasional drinking won't affect you, but prolonged, problem drinking will. "Alcoholics are especially prone to developing cataracts, because alcoholism interferes with the nutritional pathway of food to the lens, making cataract formation more likely," says Dr. Knopf. Even in alcoholics who have good diets, essential nutrients intended for the eye are diverted.

Remember: Smoke gets to your eyes. Researchers at Johns Hopkins University in Baltimore report that cigarette smokers are more likely than nonsmokers to develop cataracts. That's because toxic substances in smoke damage the lens nucleus, causing cataracts. The good news is that by quitting smoking, you *halve* your risk of developing cataracts (compared with those who continue to smoke).

Take pain relievers. British researchers report that people who take aspirin, ibuprofen (Advil) and acetaminophen (Tylenol) are *half* as likely to develop cataracts as other folks. That's because cataract formation is related to blood sugar (one reason why people with diabetes are more susceptible to cataract formation), and there's some evidence that aspirin and aspirin-like products reduce the rate at which your body uses glucose.

CHOLESTEROL CONTROL

You may have noticed that *beef* and *eggs* have become four-letter words. It's all because of cholesterol, a substance that's gotten a reputation for breaking more hearts than a high school prom queen.

But cholesterol isn't entirely bad. The human body actually needs it—and produces it—to help protect nerves and build new cells and hormones. In fact, our bodies get all the cholesterol they need by making it on their own. The trouble starts when we *add* to the cholesterol our bodies produce, which can happen when we eat the all-American diet of cheeseburgers, steaks, pizza, ice cream or any food that is or includes an animal product.

Excess cholesterol settles along arterial walls, and that excess can clog arteries and restrict blood flow, leading to angina pain, heart attack or stroke. (Cholesterol is also a leading cause of gallstones.)

If your doctor has determined that you have high levels of cholesterol in your blood, you probably have been told the importance of limiting or eliminating it—which means reducing or avoiding its only dietary sources: meat, eggs, dairy products and the foods that contain them. But here are some other ways to control your cholesterol with diet.

Stock up on vitamin E. Scientists have discovered that we have both good (high-density lipoprotein, or HDL) and bad (low-density lipoprotein, or LDL) cholesterol running through our bloodstream. Consuming 400 international units of vitamin E each day may help keep the bad cholesterol from oxidizing—an internal "rusting" process that causes the cholesterol to harden into arterial plaque, which in turn causes heart disease. Vitamin E also raises the level of good cholesterol.

"Taking vitamin E supplements helps prevent the cholesterol in your body from plaquing, so it does less damage," says Karen E. Burke, M.D., Ph.D., a dermatologist and dermatologic surgeon in New York City who has studied the various effects of vitamin E. Vitamin E is found in vegetable oils, nuts and grains, but it would be very difficult to obtain 400 international units daily from diet alone. Be sure to check with your doctor, though, before beginning a supplement program.

Add vitamin C to your menu. Other vitamins and minerals also have a beneficial effect on cholesterol. Research by Paul Jacques, Sc.D., an epidemiologist at the U.S. Department of Agriculture Human Nutrition Research Center on Aging at Tufts University in Boston, shows that people with diets high in vitamin C tend to have higher HDL levels. Vitamin C is especially beneficial when you get it from fruits and vegetables that also have a cholesterol-lowering fiber called pectin. Pectin surrounds cholesterol and helps transport it out of your digestive system before it gets into your blood. Vitamin C–rich, pectin-rich foods include citrus fruits, tomatoes, potatoes, strawberries, apples and spinach.

Eat breakfast *every* morning. Breakfast skippers tend to have higher cholesterol levels than those who start off their mornings with a bellyful, according to studies. One reason may be that breakfast skippers make up for missing the morning feast by munching on unhealthy snacks later on, suggests John L. Stanton, Ph.D., professor of food marketing at St. Joseph's University in Philadelphia.

Research also shows that those who eat ready-to-eat cereal for breakfast have lower cholesterol levels than those choosing other morning entrees.

Nibble throughout the day. One way to lower your cholesterol is simply to change how often you eat. Research has shown that large meals trigger the release of large amounts of insulin, according to David Jenkins, M.D., Ph.D., director of the Clinical Nutrition and Risk Factor Modification Center at St. Michael's Hospital at the University of Toronto. Insulin release in turn stimulates the production of an enzyme that increases cholesterol production by the liver.

Having smaller, more frequent meals (but not increasing overall calories) may limit insulin release and play a role in cholesterol control and heart disease prevention, speculates Dr. Jenkins.

Go heavy on garlic. Vampires aren't the only thing garlic keeps away. In large doses—at least seven cloves daily—this food can significantly reduce cholesterol. Of course, that's probably more garlic than most people eat in a month. To get a similar benefit, try odorless garlic pills. When people with moderately high cholesterol took four capsules a day of an odorless liquid garlic extract called Kyolic, their cholesterol levels initially rose but then fell an average of 44 points after six months, according to a research study headed by Benjamin Lau, M.D., Ph.D., at Loma Linda University School of Medicine in Loma Linda, California. You can find garlic pills at most health food stores.

Don't depend on decaf. Decaffeinated coffee actually raises LDL levels more than regular brew, so it's the worst beverage selection if you have high cholesterol, according to Dr. Jenkins. It may be because the beans used for decaf are stronger than "regular" beans. Frequent coffee drinkers (those who drink it daily) typically have a 7 percent cholesterol increase, as shown in a study at Stanford University in Stanford, California.

Gravitate toward grapes. There's a cholesterol-lowering compound in virtually all products containing grape skin, including wine, according to pomologist Leroy Creasy, Ph.D., of Cornell University College of Agriculture and Life Sciences in Ithaca, New York. You can take advantage of these cholesterol-clobbering qualities by drinking grape juice or simply eating grapes.

Reach for grapefruit. In a study conducted by James Cerda, M.D., a gastroenterologist and professor of medicine at the University of Florida Health Science Center in Gainesville, people who ate at least 1½ cups of grapefruit sections every day lowered their cholesterol over 7 percent in two months. Grapefruit is among the fruits that contain cholesterol-lowering pectin.

UNDERSTANDING CHOLESTEROL LINGO

If all this talk about good and bad cholesterol is confusing, take heart. Here's how to understand it.

Serum cholesterol is the amount of this fatty substance in your bloodstream. Your serum cholesterol is what your doctor measures in a cholesterol test. A reading *under 200* is desirable; a reading over 240 may be dangerous and is cause for concern.

Dietary cholesterol is what you eat. For instance, an egg has 213 milligrams; an apple has none. The American Heart Association recommends that you eat no more than 300 milligrams a day.

Low-density lipoprotein (LDL) is the bad cholesterol that clogs arteries. The lower your LDL, the better.

High-density lipoprotein (HDL) is the good cholesterol that scours artery walls and helps remove harmful LDL. The higher your HDL, the better.

Cook up some beans. Lima beans, kidney beans, navy beans, soybeans and other legumes can all help lower cholesterol, according to James W. Anderson, M.D., an expert in cholesterol research who is professor of medicine and clinical nutrition at the University of Kentucky College of Medicine in Lexington. The reason these high-fiber legumes are so effective is because they, too, contain pectin. The more of these beans you can eat, the greater the benefits. In one study, Dr. Anderson asked men to eat 1½ cups of cooked beans a day. The result? Their cholesterol plummeted 20 percent in just three weeks.

High-fiber diets have many other benefits too. Look for a cookbook or two that have great recipes with beans, and try to get more in your diet.

Munch a couple of carrots. Bugs Bunny's favorite entree is a boon to arteries, because carrots have plenty of cholesterol-lowering pectin. "It may be possible for people with high cholesterol to lower it 10 to 20 percent just by eating two carrots a day," says Peter D. Hoagland, Ph.D., a researcher at the U.S. Department of Agriculture Eastern Regional Research Center in Philadelphia.

Switch to olive oil. Olive oil—and certain other foods like nuts, avocados, canola oil and peanut oil—are high in still another type of fat: monounsaturated. Previously thought to have no real effect on cholesterol levels, monounsaturates may actually lower cholesterol.

Studies by cholesterol researcher Scott M. Grundy, Ph.D., at the University of Texas Southwestern Medical Center, Dallas, found that a diet high in monounsaturated fat lowered total cholesterol levels even more than a strict low-fat diet. What's more, his studies showed that monos selectively lowered the (bad) LDLs while leaving the (good) HDLs intact.

So strive for a low-fat diet, then "supplement" it with 2 or 3 tablespoons of olive oil (or an equivalent amount of other mono-rich food) each day. Just make sure you're replacing other fats with monos and not simply adding to them.

CHRONIC FATIGUE SYNDROME

I f the flu makes you feel as though you've been hit by a car, then chronic fatigue syndrome (CFS) is like getting socked by the entire General Motors assembly line. Flulike symptoms are typical of CFS—a low-grade fever, sore throat, assorted aches and pains and the kind of dead-on-your-feet fatigue that makes a slug look industrious.

But *unlike* real flu, this so-called yuppie flu just won't go away—not in days, weeks or even months; it's so bad that many people can't get out of bed, let alone hold jobs.

Doctors aren't sure what causes CFS, nor do they agree on how best to treat it. Some consider CFS a sleep disorder, since its victims often sleep *twice* as long as other people, yet still feel severely fatigued. Others think it results from stress, since CFS often strikes young high achievers who lead stressful lives but otherwise are in good health. And researchers wonder why 80 percent of CFS patients are women, most of them between the ages of 25 and 45.

While the search for some concrete answers continues, here are some of the things doctors say you should do if you're diagnosed as having CFS.

Try to stay active. Some experts heartily encourage CFS patients to exercise *lightly* each day. "It's important to stay active, even if a 50-yard walk up and down the block is all you can do comfortably," says James F. Jones, M.D., immunologist at the National Jewish Center for Immunology and Respiratory Medicine in Denver.

Jay A. Goldstein, M.D., director of the Chronic Fatigue Syndrome Institute in Anaheim Hills, California, suspects that exercise plays a key role in preventing CFS. "It's been documented that people who were in good physical condition before they got sick don't get as sick from CFS as those who weren't exercisers, and they rebound quicker."

But don't overexert yourself. "While exercise is important, you don't want to exercise to the point where you'll wind up in bed for a week afterward because you overexerted yourself," says Dr. Goldstein. "I tell people that they should exercise until they begin to perspire."

Get *mucho* magnesium. Some doctors and researchers have concluded that CFS sufferers may have abnormally low levels of magnesium in their blood. "I've noticed that about *half* of my CFS patients are also magnesium deficient," says Allan Magaziner, D.O., a Cherry Hill, New Jersey, family practitioner who specializes in nutritional therapy and preventive medicine. Good food sources of magnesium include dark green, leafy vegetables, peas, nuts and whole grains such as brown rice and soybeans.

Junk the junk food in your diet. "Another thing I've noticed is that many of my CFS patients eat way too much sugar, white flour and processed foods," adds Dr. Magaziner, who has treated more than 200 CFS patients. He recommends to his patients that they stick with well-balanced, "home-cooked" meals with plenty of fresh vegetables.

Make up for missing nutrients. Several vitamins and minerals that may be missing from processed foods can benefit CFS patients. "I tell all my patients to take a multivitamin, even if they are eating fairly good diets. It certainly can't hurt," says Dr. Goldstein.

Pay *special* attention to allergies. "Allergies in CFS patients can sometimes be very pronounced, since the immune system is activated to fight whatever is causing this illness," says James Kornish, a CFS researcher at Brigham and Women's Hospital in Boston. "If you know you are allergic to something, be careful to avoid it." And Dr. Goldstein advises against drinking red wine or eating aged cheeses, since these foods can trigger migrainelike headaches in CFS patients.

Have a *good* night's sleep. CFS patients have a greater need for sleep, and while they may get more sleep, it's not always good quality. "You aren't going to get better if you don't sleep well," says Dr. Goldstein.

Talk it out with loved ones. "It helps when family members and significant others can understand the illness, so they don't think the person is lazy or crazy," says Dr. Goldstein. "Many CFS patients feel very unsupported because they can't work and their families think they're just being lazy. Many marriages and friendships have broken up over this disease." Dr. Goldstein points out that conflict in relationships can add to stress, and additional stress only makes symptoms worse.

Air your feelings. Get help on how to deal emotionally with the disease. You can seek counseling or get support from CFS patient groups. Those patients who can maintain a positive attitude seem to cope the best.

DEPRESSION

Depression used to be such a depressing subject that people often felt compelled to fake a smile and keep their anxious, sad feelings inside.

Not anymore. Ever since researchers started to discover the mix of psychological and physical causes for this problem, depression has seemed much less mysterious and forbidding. People are acknowledging it, and talking about it, out in the open.

There are countless ways to tackle depression, from exercise to drugs to support groups. Often it's a combination of things—getting organized, learning new behaviors, becoming more self-aware—that finally breaks depression's hold.

The following tips can help you deal with life's normal ups and downs and perhaps help you bounce back faster from the downs.

Take the high road. Or the low road—it doesn't matter. Just get out there and *move.* "I tell my patients 'The odds are good to excellent that if you exercise, you will be virtually depression-free in three to five weeks,'" says psychologist Keith Johnsgard, Ph.D., professor emeritus of psychology at San Jose State University in San Jose, California, and author of *The Exercise Prescription for Depression and Anxiety.*

Studies are clear on this. The less active you are, the more likely you'll be depressed. "And a dozen or so studies show that all but the most severely depressed people who begin to exercise do as well as those who get standard psychotherapy," Dr. Johnsgard says. His exercise Rx: an hour a day of brisk walking.

What if you're too bummed out to boogie? "Get a family member or friend to come and drag you around the block a few times," he says.

Stay up to watch the sunrise. Some studies show that approximately 60 percent of depressed people who deprive themselves of a night's sleep may help thwart their symptoms, but the effects last only until the next time they sleep, says Ronald Salomon, M.D., assistant professor of psychiatry at Yale University

School of Medicine in New Haven, Connecticut. And if you use sleep deprivation for more than a night or two in one week, the mood-enhancing effects may drop off significantly, he says.

Cultivate friends. "Being able to develop and maintain intimate, supportive relationships with other people is the survival skill of the 1990s," says Ellen McGrath, Ph.D., former chairperson of the American Psychological Association's National Task Force on Women and Depression. "These relationships are critical to our health."

Realize that it takes time and effort to build these special relationships—then get to work! "Do everything and anything you can to develop the skills it takes to have quality relationships," she says. That includes learning communication skills, improving self-esteem and taking the time to be with people, Dr. McGrath says.

Know that action equals power. "Talking about your fears and anger can be helpful, but for women, it isn't enough to avert depression," Dr. McGrath says. "Taking some positive action, on the other hand, creates its own energy, which leads to a feeling of power and control." She suggests ritual actions—burning a list of worries, for instance—and real actions—such as getting organized, getting enough sleep or delegating household chores—as ways to convert uncomfortable feelings into positive action.

Tell your internal critic to take a hike. Do you have a little (or a big) voice inside you that insists nothing you do is right? That you're never going to get what you want?

"Rather than trying to get it to go away, which it never does, change your response to it," suggests Michael D. Yapko, Ph.D., a clinical psychologist in San Diego and author of *Free Yourself from Depression*. "Rather than just believing what it tells you, say to yourself 'Okay, I understand that there is this critical voice, but I don't have to listen to it.'"

People with high self-esteem also have this critical voice, Dr. Yapko says. "But they know to ignore it or at least respond to it as though what it's saying isn't true."

Don't take things so personally. "Because I don't return your phone call, you decide that I must be angry with you. That's personalizing," Dr. Yapko explains.

The problem with personalizing is that it's not a very objective way to look at things. "You jump to the first plausible conclusion, but is that the true explanation?" he asks.

A key strategy for jettisoning this kind of faulty negative thinking is to generate multiple explanations for important things that happen. "Consider a variety of possibilities and look for facts. That, at least, puts you in reality," he says.

Avoid all-or-none thinking. Do you get a C on an exam and feel like a failure? Do you miss out on a promotion at work and feel like a loser? If so, you tend to see things in black and white, with little or no gray in between. Few things in life are so extreme.

"Depressed people tend to have a low frustration tolerance," Dr. Yapko says. "They want immediate answers and immediate clarity. Typically, that's the way they've learned to be. And that's why they get depressed, because life choices are rarely clear and often ambiguous."

Learning to recognize and live with life's uncertainties is a key strategy for avoiding depression.

Try and try again—then quit. "As kids and adolescents, we have ideas of what life will bring, and sometimes we hang on to them even when life dictates that these ideas are unrealistic," says Arnold H. Gessel, M.D., a private practice psychiatrist in Broomall, Pennsylvania. Chasing elusive goals can lead to depression, he says. This is when you simply have to say "I've given it my best shot"—and give up.

Get to know yourself better. "People often get depressed when they aren't doing what they want to be doing," Dr. Yapko says. "They may want to play, for example, but feel they must always work." Fortunately, everyday life gives you the opportunity to ask yourself important, self-defining questions, he says.

"Who are you? What do you want out of life? What are the things that really matter to you? What things do you need to include in your life that are uniquely you? Make sure you build those things into your life."

Do a medicine chest shakedown. "Many drugs can cause depression," says Arthur Jacknowitz, Pharm.D., professor and chairman of clinical pharmacy at West Virginia University School of Pharmacy in Morgantown. The most likely culprits are high blood pressure medications, anti-arrhythmia drugs, prednisone and similar corticosteroids, glaucoma medications, sedatives such as Xanax and Valium, oral contraceptives and some over-the-counter drugs containing antihistamines.

"Symptoms of drug-related depression may not surface right away," Dr. Jacknowitz explains. "So even if you've been taking a medication for six months to a year and then begin to experience the blues, it could still be your medication." Discuss the problem with your doctor, he suggests. It may be possible to taper off the use of the drug or to switch to another.

DIABETES

Who'd think you can be *too* sweet? Well, it's possible. If you have diabetes, all that extra sugar (or glucose) floating around in your bloodstream can lead to trouble—nerve damage, vision loss, infections, poor circulation, kidney and heart problems, you name it. That's why it's so important to get blood sugar down to a normal level.

Normally the food we eat is converted into glucose and used or stored by the body with little problem. Circulating insulin hormone stimulates the uptake of sugar by the body's cells. But with diabetes, something goes awry. The pancreas, which is the organ responsible for producing insulin, becomes irresponsible. It either stops producing the hormone completely (Type I diabetes) or else produces too much, which leads to insulin resistance (Type II diabetes). Either way, concentration of sugar in the blood shoots sky-high.

People with Type I, or insulin-dependent, diabetes need daily insulin injections. Those with Type II, or non-insulin-dependent, diabetes—the most common form of the disease—usually don't need insulin injections. But 25 percent of them take drugs to improve sugar metabolism.

Here's what doctors are recommending to treat diabetes with diet and exercise. To determine what's appropriate for your individual situation, it's important that you check with your doctor before making changes.

Peel off some pounds. Most people with Type II diabetes are 30 to 60 pounds overweight, and for them, losing weight is often the *only* thing they have to do to get their diabetes under control, according to James Barnard, Ph.D., professor of physiological science at the University of California, Los Angeles, and consultant to the Pritikin Longevity Center in Santa Monica. Several studies point out that it's not necessary to reach your normal weight to see a big drop in blood glucose, he adds. "Ten pounds may make a difference."

But don't go to extremes. Fad diets, fasting and skipping meals don't work. Decreasing dietary fat is the best approach if you're overweight. One way is to decrease total fat to no more than 50 grams daily, says Christine Beebe, R.D., director of the diabetes program at St. James Hospital in Chicago Heights, Illinois, and chairman of the Council on Nutritional Science and Metabolism for the American Diabetes Association.

Get moving. "Spend 45 minutes to one hour taking a good brisk walk every day," Dr. Barnard says. "It helps normalize body weight, and it helps correct insulin resistance, which is the main problem in Type II diabetes."

Stay regular as clockwork. "If you take insulin or insulin-stimulating drugs, as some people with Type II diabetes do, exercising at the same time three to six days a week for the same amount of time can be helpful," says Beebe. "That makes it easier to control your blood sugar."

If you *don't* exercise every day, pay particular attention on the days that you do. "You may need to cut your insulin dose 30 to 50 percent," Beebe says.

Change flab to firm. Muscle building and weight training can play an important role in diabetes control. "Having more muscle and less fat improves insulin sensitivity, so less insulin is needed to respond to sugar in the blood," says Bruce W. Craig, Ph.D., associate director of exercise science at Ball State University in Muncie, Indiana. "It means people with diabetes may be able to reduce their insulin intake and still handle the sugar in their blood—their glucose—effectively." Once you get your doctor's okay, join a health club that has weight-training equipment. Ask the club for professional instruction before you begin.

Cut the fat. At the Pritikin Longevity Center, the diet is carefully designed to cut out fat. Meals at the center are super low in fat, with less than 10 percent of calories from fat, 10 to 15 percent from protein and 75 to 80 percent from carbohydrates (such as veggies and fruits). What does that look like on your plate? Grains and beans, vegetables, fruits, nonfat milk and an occasional piece of fish or fowl. The good part is that except for the meat, you get to eat as much as you want. Adds Dr. Barnard: "Any reduction in fat is going to help your diabetes and your overall health."

Be especially particular about breakfast. "There's some evidence that those with diabetes have a harder time with carbohydrates in the morning, when insulin resistance is greatest," Beebe says. Reducing carbohydrates and adding protein might be your best bet. Try skim milk and oatmeal, for example, or an occasional poached egg with a slice of whole wheat toast, or cottage cheese and crackers. Check your blood glucose before lunch to see how you're doing. The next day you can adjust your food intake further, if necessary.

Eat smaller meals more often. The diabetic body can handle smaller meals more easily because the smaller the meal, the less insulin is needed to handle the glucose influx from each meal, says registered dietitian Marion Franz, M.S., R.D., vice president of nutrition at the International Diabetes Center in Minneapolis, Minnesota. Less glucose equals less insulin equals more constant blood sugar levels. Some diabetes meal plans call for three meals a day or three small meals plus one or two small snacks between meals. Franz says she favors more actual meals because "often if people go too long between meals they get so hungry they can't control what they eat at the next meal." She also recommends snacks like a piece of fruit or a couple of crackers between meals.

Eat food with fiber. Natural fiber in food has been found to have a host of beneficial effects for everyone. That goes double for people with diabetes. The American Diabetes Association advises you to gradually head for 40 grams a day. Whole wheat products, barley, oats, legumes, vegetables, and fruit are the best sources of fiber, as well as essential nutrients.

One possible benefit fiber provides diabetics is lower cholesterol levels. "The water-soluble fibers found in legumes, oats, barley, and fruit, when eaten in a low-fat diet, have been shown to lower blood fat levels," Franz says. "Because they form a gel in the gastrointestinal tract," they may also cause the energy (sugar) in food to be absorbed at a slower rate, giving your insulin a chance to keep your blood sugar on a more even keel.

Fiber also helps keep you from feeling hungry. "I think one of the main benefits of fiber is that it adds bulk to the diet," Franz says. "For Type II people who are trying to control their weight and so are on restricted calories, bulk lets people feel fuller."

Besides giving you that pleasantly satiated feeling, fiber foods are good for you. "They're often high in important vitamins and minerals," Franz says.

Treat booze like fat. Alcohol is high in empty calories. "We recommend that people keep their alcohol consumption down to fewer than three drinks a week," Dr. Barnard says.

Chrome-plate your diet. Make sure you're getting enough chromium, a trace mineral that helps normalize blood sugar levels—high *or* low (it gives insulin a boost). In fact, in some cases, chromium may help prevent Type II diabetes.

Studies show that typical Americans do not get nearly enough chromium in their diets, even when calorie intake is fairly high, says Richard A. Anderson, Ph.D., a biochemist at the U.S. Department of Agriculture Human Nutrition Research Center in Beltsville, Maryland. "Regardless of how you cut the cards, you're not getting enough chromium in your diet," he says. "Even diets designed by dietitians don't provide nearly enough chromium."

His suggestion: Take a chromium supplement in addition to a balanced multivitamin/mineral supplement. "In our studies, we use 200 micrograms a day, and that works very well," says Dr. Anderson. But check with your doctor before taking any supplemental dose.

Honor the East when you eat. Laboratory tests show that cinnamon and turmeric (the golden spice used in curry

SELF-TREATMENT FOR
MILD HYPOGLYCEMIA

Hypoglycemia occurs when blood sugar drops too low. Because keeping their blood sugar at normal levels requires quite a balancing act, diabetics are particularly prone to hypoglycemia. People with adult-onset diabetes usually get hypoglycemia from skipping or delaying meals, or from unplanned-for strenuous exercise.

Symptoms of mild hypoglycemia include numbness in the mouth, cool wet skin, a fluttering feeling in the chest and hunger.

To treat it yourself, says American Diabetes Association past president Karl Sussman, M.D., associate chief of staff for research and development at the Veterans Administration Hospital in Denver, "you need to take some form of sugar that's readily available." Drink something sweet like orange juice or soda, or eat a candy bar, he says, and be ready for it by carrying candy or mints with you.

dishes) *triple* the ability of insulin to metabolize glucose, says Dr. Anderson. "There's a long history of spices being used in the treatment of diabetes, especially in India, Pakistan and China," he says. If cooking is your thing, get a couple of oriental cookbooks that have tasty recipes using these spices. And look for curry dishes when you dine out.

DIVERTICULOSIS

It's okay to *act* refined at the dinner table, but when you *eat* that way, don't expect your colon to always keep its good manners. Living off refined or overly processed foods and other low-fiber fare puts so much pressure on colon walls (as you try to pass hard, dry stools) that they may develop tiny pouches called diverticula. This results in gas, cramping, severe indigestion and even diarrhea or constipation as these pouches become inflamed.

In a worst-case scenario, feces can get stuck in the pouches, causing internal bleeding and serious infection. This condition, called diverticul*itis*, occurs in only about 5 percent of cases and usually requires surgery. But there's a minor form of this problem called diverticul*osis* that's far more common than the version requiring surgery. Many people have learned after seeing their doctor that they can treat the condition themselves. And here's how.

Feast on fiber. "A high-fiber diet is the answer for treating diverticulosis," says gastroenterologist Alex Aslan, M.D., a staff physician at North Bay Medical Center in Fairfield, California. "That helps normalize the stool and reduce the pressure on your colon that's causing the problem in the first place."

To get more fiber, limit consumption of processed foods. Instead, always try to eat more whole-grain breads, grains and cereals, beans, fruits and vegetables.

You can also benefit from taking a psyllium product such as Metamucil each day. Psyllium is a natural high-fiber ingredient that can help speed movement in the intestines. Just follow the directions on the package.

Be sure to increase your fiber intake slowly, says Stephen B. Hanauer, M.D., professor of medicine in the Section of Gastroenterology at the University of Chicago Medical Center. And don't give up if you develop some gas symptoms—that's a normal introduction to a high-fiber diet.

Wet your whistle. While most doctors recommend that everyone should drink no less than six glasses of water a day, it's especially important if you have diverticulosis. Liquids are an important partner to fiber in softening stools and combating constipation, which is associated with diverticulosis, says Samuel Klein, M.D., associate professor of medicine in the Division of Gastroenterology and in the Division of Human Nutrition at the University of Texas Medical School at Galveston.

Don't smoke. "Besides being the single worst thing you can do to your overall health, smoking is terrible for your intestines," says Dr. Hanauer. "What smoking does is increase motility in your intestines, but the nicotine decreases the blood supply. This causes or increases your cramps."

Coffee, no; alcohol, yes, but . . . You should also limit or avoid coffee, since caffeine can cause diarrhea, while chemicals in coffee beans may cause cramping, adds Dr. Aslan. But alcohol in small quantities—no more than two drinks daily—may actually *help* by relaxing colon spasms, says Marvin M. Schuster, M.D., chief of the Department of Digestive Diseases at Francis Scott Key Medical Center in Baltimore.

Hit the road. "Running very clearly stimulates bowel activity and is very useful to anyone who is irregular," says Dr. Hanauer. Other forms of aerobic activity such as swimming, cycling and fast walking also help by improving blood flow through the colon.

ECZEMA AND DERMATITIS

Some people know it as eczema. Others know it as dermatitis, the newer classification for any of several different types of skin inflammation. But anyone who's ever had these bothersome skin rashes—characterized by red, oozing, scaly and itchy patches—has probably referred to it by names that would make a sailor blush.

That's a lot of @$*&#*! and even more scratching, since untold tens of millions suffer some form of eczema/dermatitis each year. There are *at least* five different "groupings" of these skin irritations. The symptoms for each group are a little different, but all have one thing in common—misery.

Get clean—without soaps. "The smartest thing you can do is to use the most gentle cleanser you can find—definitely not regular toilet soaps," advises Nelson Lee Novick, M.D., associate clinical professor of dermatology at Mount Sinai School of Medicine in New York City. "They clean just as well and are much less irritating to the skin. You'll find them in your drugstore labeled as cleansing 'bars' or 'cakes,' or you can go with a liquid cleanser that's labeled as 'nonirritating,' such as Moisturel Sensitive Skin Cleanser." The same goes for shampoos: "Use baby shampoo or other mild types," suggests Dr. Novick.

Heal with oatmeal. "Oatmeal baths made from powders such as Aveeno provide effective but temporary relief from the itching of eczema and dermatitis," says Stephen M. Purcell, D.O., chairman of the Department of Dermatology at Philadelphia College of Osteopathic Medicine and assistant clinical professor at Hahnemann University School of Health Sciences in Philadelphia.

Relieve the itch with ice. "An ice pack made by putting ice cubes in a plastic bag and placing it on the itchy area makes an inexpensive and effective itch fighter," adds Michael Ramsey,

M.D., a dermatologist and clinical instructor of dermatology at Baylor College of Medicine in Houston. Make sure that the ice pack is wrapped in a towel.

And milk is "udderly" effective. For weeping eczema, which "oozes," a compress of cold milk is another way to soothe itchy skin, says John F. Romano, M.D., a dermatologist and clinical assistant professor of medicine at The New York Hospital–Cornell Medical Center in New York City. Pour some cold milk onto a gauze pad or thin piece of cotton and apply it to the skin for about three minutes. Resoak the cloth and reapply at least two more times for three-minute soaks. Repeat several times a day, but make sure to rinse your skin in cool water after each application, because the milk will smell.

Avoid *most* antiperspirants. The active "drying" ingredients found in most antiperspirants—aluminum chloride, aluminum sulfate and zirconium chlorohydrates—are too irritating to those with dry, sensitive skin, cautions Howard Donsky, M.D., associate professor of medicine at the University of Toronto, and author of *Beauty Is Skin Deep*. "I recommend that people use an antiseptic soap such as Dial or Zest. Also, Tom's of Maine Natural Deodorant is a very gentle product."

But stay dry and odor-free. Baking soda is an excellent alternative to commercially sold antiperspirants, adds Dr. Novick. Besides being less expensive, it absorbs excess moisture without irritating dry or sensitive skin.

Keep nails short and clean. Short nails are less effective at scratching—and you don't want to scratch. "Not only will scratching aggravate your skin, but it can break and damage it, contributing to secondary bacterial infections," says Jerome Z. Litt, M.D., a dermatologist and assistant clinical professor of dermatology at Case Western Reserve University School of Medicine in Cleveland. Clean, short nails are less likely to irritate or cause infection in case you do scratch.

Sit on your hands. In Sweden, where the cold winter air makes skin incredibly dry, researchers have been very successful in teaching eczema patients "antiscratching therapy." In the first of two sessions, patients were taught to press firmly on the itchy area for one minute whenever they had an urge to scratch—and then immediately move their hands to their thighs or to an object. In the second session, patients avoided the itchy area entirely—instead moving their hands *directly* to their thighs or an object. After four weeks, patients given this therapy and a hydrocortisone cream had *twice* the improvement, compared with those given only the cream.

Humidify your surroundings. As with winter itch or any form of dry skin, "anything you can do to add moisture to the air is going to help," says Dr. Novick. "I recommend either buying a cold-air humidifier or placing shallow pans of water near radiators and on wood stoves to add humidity."

Keep showers extra short. "Your showers should last about three minutes—and *no longer* than five minutes," adds Dr. Novick. "The only baths you should take are oatmeal baths, because baths encourage you to stay in the tub longer—and water *adds* to your dryness. Hot water is especially drying, so keep the water as cool as possible."

And use only your fingertips to wash—*not* washcloths or sponges—and then pat yourself dry.

Don't forget your emollients. Those containing urea or lactic acid are best for relieving itching, says Hillard H. Pearlstein, M.D., assistant clinical professor of dermatology at Mount Sinai School of Medicine in New York City. Carmol 10, Carmol 20 and Ultra Mide 25 contain urea, and Lac-Hydrin Five contains lactic acid.

Wash once, rinse twice. Laundry detergents are another no-no, because these powerful soaps are especially irritating, adds Dr. Purcell. "It's wise to double-rinse your laundry to make sure the detergent rinses out and won't come in contact with your skin."

DITCH THE ITCH

Here are some other things that you should avoid if you're prone to eczema.

- Baby lotions. The added fragrances and lanolins are common causes of skin allergies, says John F. Romano, M.D., a dermatologist and clinical assistant professor of medicine at The New York Hospital–Cornell Medical Center in New York City.
- Colored toilet paper and tissues. Their dyes are irritating to many, so when it's time to wipe, stick with white, advises Howard Donsky, M.D., associate professor of medicine at the University of Toronto.
- Stuffed animals. Fuzzy and furry toys and pillows can bother those with sensitive skin, says Jerome Z. Litt, M.D., assistant clinical professor of dermatology at Case Western Reserve University School of Medicine in Cleveland.
- Real animals. Sorry, but man's best friend—particularly long-haired breeds—is anything but friendly to those with eczema, adds Dr. Litt. He advises keeping dogs and cats outdoors—at least until your skin improves.
- Fake fingernails. They cause very real dermatitis in some people. Dr. Donsky blames the problem on acrylics in some artificial and sculptured fingernail products.
- Live Christmas trees. Metal trees may not be as appealing, but Dr. Litt says that they're less allergenic to eczema sufferers.
- Quick changes in air temperature. Quickly going from a nice, warm room into the cold outdoors, or vice versa, plays havoc with your skin, says Dr. Donsky. Spending some "in-between" time in a mudroom or wearing layers of cotton clothing—and peeling them off slowly—can help.
- Metallic jewelry. If you're prone to nickel allergies—the most common form of contact dermatitis—then avoid watchbands, earrings and jewelry that cause a skin reaction. Buying earrings? Look for earring posts that are stainless steel.

Don't use dryer sheets. "Some of the chemicals in fabric-softening dryer sheets remain on the skin and can be irritating to people with eczema," says Rodney Basler, M.D., a dermatologist and assistant professor of internal medicine at the University of Nebraska Medical Center in Omaha. "However, fabric softeners you add to the washing machine don't seem to irritate."

Don't be a fool if you use a pool. "If you do a lot of swimming in chlorine-filled pools, you have to take even more precautions," advises Dr. Novick. "*Immediately* after leaving the pool, rinse off your body in cool water and apply a moisturizer."

Buy American when it comes to cosmetics. The general rule is, avoid cosmetics if you're bothered by eczema or dermatitis. But if you must wear them, buy American. That's because some cosmetics made in Japan, Italy, France and other foreign countries contain formaldehyde, which can cause allergic dermatitis in many people, says Mary Ellen Brademas, M.D., chief of dermatology at St. Vincent's Hospital and assistant clinical professor of dermatology at New York University Medical Center, both in New York City.

Relax. "Stress is a definite contributing factor in eczema as well as other skin conditions," says Dr. Basler. "If you are feeling stressed out or are particularly worried about something, it will only aggravate your condition."

EMPHYSEMA

A typical set of lungs contains about 300 million tiny, elastic air sacs that, with every breath, add oxygen to the blood and remove carbon dioxide. Emphysema occurs when the elasticity in these sacs changes and they enlarge and rupture—making it impossible to fully exhale.

Father Time can take some of the blame, since most people experience a change in lung elasticity as they age (though usually not enough to cause serious problems). And maybe you can cast some blame on genes, too, as a small percentage of folks *inherit* a protein deficiency that causes emphysema. But if you want to point the finger at culprit number one, it's tobacco: Most emphysema strikes long-term smokers and is a direct result of smoking.

Emphysema is serious business. It can make breathing difficult and simple chores nearly impossible. It also increases the risk of heart disease by interfering with the passage of blood through the lungs. For many people, even eating becomes difficult. But even though it's usually irreversible, here's what you can do to deemphasize emphysema and breathe easier.

Munch a bunch. Since people with emphysema cannot fully exhale, the lungs enlarge with trapped air. The enlarged lungs push down into the abdomen, leaving less room for the stomach to expand—making eating uncomfortable.

"Many people with emphysema find it's much better to eat many smaller meals instead of three large ones," says Barry Make, M.D., director of pulmonary rehabilitation at the National Jewish Center for Immunology and Respiratory Medicine in Denver. "When you eat a large meal, it puts more pressure on the stomach and pushes up the diaphragm, which makes it more difficult to breathe. Besides eating a lot of little meals, it's also important to take small bites, to eat slowly and to chew your food well, which will make it easier on your breathing."

"A lot of people with emphysema lose weight or have trouble keeping weight on because eating can become so difficult," adds Mark J. Rosen, M.D., chief of the Division of Pulmonary and

Critical Care Medicine at Beth Israel Medical Center in New York City. "You want to avoid weight loss, so be sure to eat enough."

Profit from produce. Some of the most advantageous eats you can have are fresh fruits and vegetables high in vitamin C and beta-carotene. "Some evidence suggests that vitamin C and beta-carotene may help protect against a decline in lung function," says Joel Schwartz, Ph.D., an epidemiologist and senior scientist at the Environmental Protection Agency in Washington, D.C. "It may be a very minimal effect in those with emphysema, but eating foods rich in these nutrients certainly won't hurt and may help."

Good sources of vitamin C include citrus fruits, strawberries and other fruits, as well as peppers and broccoli. Beta-carotene is abundant in sweet potatoes, squash, carrots and other fruits and vegetables with a yellowish orange color.

Breathe from your diaphragm. This is the most efficient way to breathe. Babies do it naturally. If you watch them, you'll see their bellies rise and fall with each breath.

Not sure whether you're breathing from your diaphragm or your chest? Francisco Perez, Ph.D., a clinical assistant professor of neurology and physical medicine at Baylor College of Medicine, tells his patients to lie down, put City of Houston–size phone directories on their bellies and watch what happens to them when they breathe.

Keep those airways open. You can strengthen your breathing muscles if you blow out slowly through pursed lips for 30 minutes a day, says Henry Gong, M.D., professor of medicine at the University of California, Los Angeles, and associate chief of the Pulmonary Division at UCLA Medical Center. Try to exhale twice as long as it took you to breathe in. This will help you rid the lungs of stale air, so fresh air can get in.

You can also buy a device from your pharmacy that offers resistance when you blow against it. "It looks like a little plastic mouthpiece with a ring on the end," says pulmonary specialist Robert Sandhaus, M.D., Ph.D., consultant for the National

Jewish Center for Immunology and Respiratory Medicine and other health facilities in Denver. "When you turn the ring, the opening at the mouthpiece changes size. You start with the largest opening, take a deep breath in and blow out. Once you master one setting, you move on to another one."

Stop smoking *now*! "When you stop smoking, you slow the deterioration of your lungs, and that's probably the best thing you can do once you've been diagnosed with emphysema," says Dr. Rosen. "Besides that, you will boost your feeling of well-being. And you'll be able to exercise longer, which will improve your comfort in breathing."

Failing to quit, on the other hand, speeds the deterioration of your lungs. It's also wise to avoid any exposure to secondhand smoke as well as any substances that may trigger allergies.

Get your heart pumping. "Aerobic exercise is very important for people with emphysema because it strengthens the heart and can help improve your breathing," says Dr. Rosen. "Walking is probably the best thing you can do, and you should try to do it every day."

Although you'll probably tire quickly, try to slowly build your endurance so that you can walk for about 20 minutes at least three days a week. Riding a stationary bicycle, swimming and participating in low-impact aerobics classes are also good, adds Dr. Make.

Build your body, too. What good are bulging biceps when you have trouble breathing? "The muscles in your shoulders, arms and upper chest comprise one of the two muscle groups that participate in breathing," says Dr. Make. (The other is the diaphragm.) Whether it's doing some simple exercises while holding wrist or hand weights or starting a full-fledged weight-training program, anything you can do to build your upper body strength will help your breathing. But make sure you breathe correctly while pumping iron: Exhale through pursed lips as you lift, and inhale as you relax.

Dress in the baggy look. Wearing clothing that fits loosely around your chest and abdomen allows plenty of room for them to expand freely, keeping breathing more comfortable. You might want to try suspenders instead of a belt, a camisole instead of a bra and going without a girdle.

Don't isolate yourself socially. "You need to avoid generalizing about the shortness of breath," says Robert Teague, M.D., clinical assistant professor of medicine at Baylor College of Medicine in Houston. "Some emphysema sufferers think, 'Well, I probably can't do this.' Because they're scared they might get out somewhere and get short of breath, they quit going places they'd normally enjoy." Don't let it isolate you.

Pace yourself. "The other thing emphysema sufferers have to learn to do is to take their own time," says Dr. Teague. "They really can do what they want to do but they have to do it at their own pace. That is not an easy thing to do, to learn to walk slower."

Work smarter. Little things can make a big difference. Can you rearrange your work spaces so you can get more done with less effort? What about setting your table with dishes directly from the drying rack instead of putting them away?

The American Lung Association also suggests that you obtain a three-shelf utility cart to help you with your housework. Small efficiencies like these pay you back with extra energy.

GALLSTONES

Think of your gallbladder as a kind of storage tank for your liver. It collects bile, a cholesterol-rich fluid secreted by the liver. When you eat something fatty, your small intestine sends out a biochemical message to the gallbladder—"Hey, squirt out some bile!" The bile interacts with the food, helping to break it down into digestible bits.

Think of gallstones as sand or pebbles in the storage tank. Gallstones form when there is too much cholesterol or pigment in the bile. They start out as tiny globules but can snowball to the size of an egg.

Lots of times, gallstones don't cause any problems at all. People may not even realize they have them until they show up on an x-ray or during an ultrasound examination. When gallstones do cause pain, it's usually because one has gotten stuck in a duct, blocking the flow of bile. If that happens, you'll have steady, severe pain in the upper abdomen that lasts at least 20 minutes but may continue up to four miserable hours. You may also feel pain between the shoulder blades or in the right shoulder. Nausea and vomiting are common, too.

Pain-producing gallstones sometimes pass through the duct or drop back into the gallbladder. The pain and the problem are temporarily on hold. When they get stuck in a duct for long, though, they can cause serious problems.

Once you have pain-producing gallstones, you may be able to tame your symptoms by losing weight and going on a moderately low-fat diet, says Henry Pitt, M.D., director of the Gallstone and Biliary Disease Center at Johns Hopkins Hospital in Baltimore.

"Usually the symptoms don't go away, and you may run into complications," he adds. "So your doctor will probably recommend that your gallbladder be removed."

But if you still have a gallbladder and it's giving you gallstone problems, here's what doctors suggest to minimize symptoms.

Shed those few extra pounds. When it comes to developing gallstones, even slightly overweight people have twice the risk of people at their ideal weight. And seriously overweight people run a sixfold risk. Your doctor can check a weight/height chart to determine your ideal weight. If you're overweight, plan a change of diet and exercise to bring down your weight.

But do it gradually. Dropping weight too fast (more than a pound a week) actually increases your chances of developing gallstones, which can form within four to six months of beginning a weight-loss program. So stick with a weight-loss program that will let you reduce slowly and steadily, Dr. Pitt recommends.

Avoid no-fat diets. Virtually fat-free weight-loss diets seem to pose a particularly high risk for gallstone formation, according to several studies.

Why? An extremely low-fat diet (below 20 percent of calories from fat) allows bile to sit and concentrate in the gallbladder, explains Stanley Heshka, Ph.D., a research associate at the Obesity Research Center at St. Luke's–Roosevelt Hospital Center in New York City. Dietary fat stimulates the gallbladder to expel its contents, which reduces the concentration of cholesterol and pigments. "Research suggests that a weight-loss diet of at least 1,200 calories, with 20 percent of calories from fat, may offer protection from gallstones," he says.

But don't go overboard on the fat. Although data are conflicting, many doctors suspect a diet high in saturated fat can contribute to gallstone problems as well as to weight gain, a risk in itself. So stay away from foods that are very high in saturated fat, such as butter, highly processed foods, marbled meats and products containing palm or coconut oils.

Better not count on old-time "cures." Old-time remedies, which involve a three-day fast followed by a whopping dose of olive oil and fruit juice, are said to stimulate your gallbladder so vigorously that it spews out any stones. Some people say they actually see the stones pass in the form of greenish blobs when they try this remedy.

"I am not convinced this works," says Andrew Weil, M.D., associate director of the Division of Social Perspectives in Medicine of the College of Medicine at the University of Arizona in Tucson. "It's possible that the greenish blobs are actually residues of the olive oil, not stones."

Trying this remedy may also increase your risk of a major gallbladder attack, with the possibility of stones lodging in the bile ducts, says Johnson Thistle, M.D., professor of medicine at the Mayo Clinic in Rochester, Minnesota.

Cut the cholesterol. Not only can diets high in cholesterol lead to weight gain, the cholesterol itself also may be a problem. At Johns Hopkins, prairie dogs fed large amounts of cholesterol began to develop gallstones in just a few weeks. "The fact that we're so easily able to cause gallstones in the animals makes me think that cholesterol probably is one of many factors responsible," Dr. Pitt says.

However, these findings relate only to prairie dogs, he stresses. Further studies are needed to determine if people are similarly affected. But since diets high in cholesterol are known to contribute to *other* health problems—high blood pressure, for example, and strokes and heart attacks—cutting the cholesterol is just good sense.

Put some fish on the grill. When the prairie dogs at Johns Hopkins were fed fish oil along with their high-cholesterol feed, gallstones failed to develop, Dr. Pitt says. Again, it's too early to tell if fish oil will have a similar protective effect in people, but adding a little fish to your diet certainly can't hurt. Mackerel, salmon and tuna are among the types highest in fish oil.

GASTRITIS

T he pain started when he moved from Tulsa to Albuquerque in the early 1980s, John remembers. Perhaps it was the Southwest's spicy foods, or the cigarettes he smoked, or the late nights spent in clubs. Even stress seemed to fan the smoldering coal in his chest into burning flames.

The first few times it happened, John didn't worry about it at all. "I figured it was just a little indigestion. I'd just take an antacid after lunch, and it would usually start feeling better." Eventually, though, the burning pain in his gut started coming on more often, and he started to worry a little. Then he started to worry some more—enough to get him to ask his doctor: "Is there something wrong with my gut?"

GUT TROUBLE

What John called indigestion his doctor called gastritis—a painful but rarely serious inflammation of the stomach's lining. In fact, just about everyone suffers from occasional bouts of indigestion or heartburn, says Frank L. Lanza, M.D., clinical professor of gastroenterology at Houston's Baylor College of Medicine. For most people, it doesn't amount to more than a few minutes of discomfort every now and then. But for some people like John, any number of things can bring it on—and bring it on often.

Dr. Lanza says gastritis can be brought on by several things: heavy drinking, certain medications, spicy or acidic foods or just too many tacos—or pizza, hot dogs or egg rolls—at lunch. And it's most unpredictable. It sometimes causes painful flare-ups for hours, days or weeks at a time. Occasionally gastritis will indicate a more serious problem, such as an ulcer. But in most cases, Dr. Lanza says, gastritis is nothing more than an irritated stomach getting even.

"People come in with heartburn, with bloating and discomfort, with indigestion and dyspepsia," Dr. Lanza says. "We do all the tests and find nothing wrong except a little redness in the stomach. So you say, 'Ah, they've got gastritis.' It's a diagnosis of exclusion."

The good news about gastritis is that the symptoms can disappear as quickly as they come on. In fact, the stomach can recover from almost everything, says Dr. Lanza, including all the hot tamales John wolfed down while he lived in New Mexico. When he left the state (and its spicy cuisine), he said goodbye to his daily indigestion. Here's what you can try to help get rid of yours.

Take the acid test. As John can attest, antacids almost always work at relieving the pain. As their name suggests, antacids work by neutralizing stomach acids, which gives the inflamed stomach lining a chance to heal.

Most doctors agree that liquid antacids are more effective than tablets. Take 1 or 2 teaspoonfuls when symptoms flare.

Go on the milk wagon. At one time, doctors thought milk soothed a sore stomach. But now they know better. Milk actually *increases* the acid in the stomach. "As soon as milk's buffering effect is gone—that takes 20 to 30 minutes—the acid will just be roaring," Dr. Lanza says.

This doesn't mean you have to give up milk forever just because you have gastritis, doctors say. You can drink low-fat or skim milk, which should be easier on your insides than whole milk. But when symptoms are flaring, it's best to avoid it altogether. Reach for water instead.

Try a new painkiller. More than most drugs, aspirin is hard on your stomach, Dr. Lanza says. "Generally, people who take the enteric-coated aspirin have less gastritis than the people who take plain aspirin," he says. He also recommends that people take aspirin with meals because food in the stomach acts as a natural buffer. Or ask your doctor about aspirin substitutes such as acetaminophen.

Cut the fat. No matter what you eat, your stomach churns out acid to digest it. The bigger the meal, the more acid it produces. And when you eat foods high in fats, your stomach produces even more acid. That's good for digestion; it isn't good for gastritis. "For people with chronic indigestion, I put them on a low-fat diet," Dr. Lanza says. It's also better to eat smaller meals more often, he says, than to pack in a day's worth at one sitting.

Avoid acidic foods. If you ever tried to eat an orange when you had a mouth ulcer, you know it can sting like crazy. Well, acidic foods can also be tough on your digestive tract. If eating oranges, lemons, limes or tomatoes gives you grief, look for less painful ways to get your vitamin C—in peas, for example, and broccoli and brussels sprouts.

Change your bad habits. If wassail makes your stomach wail, try celebrating with softer drinks. Dr. Lanza always advises people with gastritis to drink less alcohol, stop smoking cigarettes and avoid coffee (especially black) and other caffeinated drinks.

SEEKING SOMETHING STRONGER

For most cases of gastritis, these self-help measures should help you stay symptom-free, says Dr. Lanza. If, however, you find you're taking seven or eight doses of antacids a day and not getting much relief, it could be a sign of something more serious, such as an ulcer. You should make an appointment to see your doctor.

Even if you don't have an ulcer, your doctor may decide that what you need is stronger medication. A prescription ulcer medication such as cimetidine (Tagamet), which reduces the quantity of acid in your stomach, can be used to relieve gastritis, says Dr. Lanza. Some people take anti-ulcer drugs *and* antacids, a combination that seems quite effective, he says.

But gastritis can be controlled. Just ask John. After letting up on the drinking, giving up smoking and forgoing overly spicy foods, John says his stomach pain rarely returns.

But John admits he'll always have to be careful what he eats. "I love orange juice, and grapefruit juice, too, but sometimes they kill me—they absolutely kill me."

GLAUCOMA

To anyone who has eye damage from glaucoma, the world is viewed through a long, narrow tunnel.

Chronic glaucoma—the most common type—has been called the "sneak thief of sight." Slowly and painlessly, fluid begins to build up in the eyeball, creating excessive pressure. The delicate nerves inside the eye—nerves that carry visual signals to the brain—are damaged by the pressure. As nerve damage continues, sight deteriorates to the point where you literally have tunnel vision. Unfortunately, unless the pressure is relieved, someone with glaucoma can lose their sight completely.

If you have glaucoma, your doctor probably has already put you on prescription eyedrops to lower the pressure in the eye.

Once on medications, you require routine eye exams two to three times a year to ensure that the damage has stopped. It's the best way to protect your sight. But in between, here's what doctors say you can do for yourself.

Don't skimp on your eyedrops. "To control glaucoma, you must take your medication every day for life, so stick to your schedule," says Kevin Greenidge, M.D., director of glaucoma services at Metropolitan Hospital Center and a member of the glaucoma service at the New York Eye and Ear Infirmary, both in New York City. If you've been advised to use your eyedrops twice daily, it means every 12 hours, says Dr. Greenidge. Four times a day means every 6 hours. But don't double up if you miss a dose, he cautions. If the doses are too large, the medication could cause blurred vision or other side effects.

Close off the drain. You can increase the effectiveness of eyedrops by pulling down your bottom eyelid, inserting the drops and then pressing your finger against the tear duct in the inner corner of your eye, says Jack Holladay, M.D., professor of ophthalmology at the University of Texas Medical School at Houston. "When you close off the drain, you prevent the medicine from going into your nose and eventually into your bloodstream, where it can cause side effects," says Dr. Holladay. Then close your eyes for two minutes, he adds. This allows the drug to be completely absorbed.

Avoid eyedrops containing cortisone. Cortisone interferes with the flow of fluid in the eyeball. As a result, it can boost pressure in the eye, according to George Spaeth, M.D., director of glaucoma services at Wills Eye Hospital and professor of ophthalmology at Jefferson Medical College of Thomas Jefferson University, both in Philadelphia.

Choose medicines with care. "If you're farsighted, talk to your doctor before using products such as Contac," says Dr. Spaeth. In some farsighted people, the area where fluid drains from the eye may be quite narrow, he says. Decongestants and antihistamines (such as Contac) dilate the pupil, narrowing the drainage canal even further. So you might risk a dangerous buildup of pressure if you take these medications.

Pedal daily to prevent pressure buildup. "Our studies showed that when people who were at risk for glaucoma cycled for a half-hour three times a week for ten weeks, they reduced the pressure in their eyes," says Linn Goldberg, M.D., associate professor of medicine and director of the General Medicine Clinics and Human Performance Laboratory at the Oregon Health Sciences University in Portland. In fact, the study showed that this cycling routine was just as effective as glaucoma drugs. "Heightened pressure inside the eye is to glaucoma what high blood pressure is to heart disease," says Dr. Goldberg. "If you can control the pressure, you can prevent some aspects of the disease." But just because you take up cycling doesn't mean you can drop your drops, cautions Dr. Goldberg. Any change in treatment requires a doctor's okay.

Take vitamin C and see. There is evidence that very high doses of vitamin C relieve eye pressure and may also help improve the visual field, according to Jay Cohen, O.D., associate professor

CHECK OUT THIS SIGHT TEST

Only an eye exam by an ophthalmologist (M.D.) can tell you whether you have early glaucoma. But you should also be alert to any changes in vision such as blurriness or "blanked-out" sight, says George Spaeth, M.D., director of glaucoma services at Wills Eye Hospital and professor of ophthalmology at Jefferson Medical College of Thomas Jefferson University, both in Philadelphia. He's developed this self-test to help you spot warning signs between eye exams.

Sit about a foot away from a large TV set tuned to a channel that has nothing but "snow"—random, blurred spots or lines. Close your left eye and look at the center of the screen with your right eye. Are any areas of the screen blanked out, washed out or less visible? Pay particular attention to the upper left-hand side of the screen: If you have trouble seeing that area, your vision loss may be caused by glaucoma. Repeat with the other eye to find out whether you've lost any vision on that side. If this quick test shows any sight loss, don't wait for your next regular eye exam. Call an ophthalmologist right away.

of optometry at the State University of New York College of Optometry in New York City. However, the amount of vitamin C in those studies was too high for practical use. "It appears that vitamin C may help draw fluid out of the eye in some way," says Dr. Cohen.

Dr. Cohen has his glaucoma patients take a maximum of 1,000 milligrams a day. "That amount can't hurt, and it could help," he says. Before trying vitamin therapy, however, get the okay from your doctor.

GOUT

O nce known as the "kings' disease" because it almost always afflicted the well heeled, this form of arthritis is an equal opportunity deployer: It delivers a *royal* pain to the toe, knee and other joints.

You'll qualify for gout if your kidneys lose some of their ability to flush away excess amounts of a by-product called uric acid. When uric acid crystallizes, it lodges in the joints, causing more than a crystal's worth of pain. "Think of what happens when you put too much sugar in a glass of iced tea," says Jeffrey R. Lisse, M.D., director of the Division of Rheumatology at the University of Texas Medical Branch in Galveston. "The sugar will dissolve up to a point, and the remaining crystals pile up at the bottom."

When that occurs, the joint can get hot, swollen and tender. Sometimes the pain is so bad that it can actually wake you from a sound sleep. "Gout occurs sporadically, but it hits like gangbusters, often in the middle of the night," says Paul Caldron, D.O., a clinical rheumatologist and researcher at the Arthritis Center in Phoenix. "We're talking about pain so intense that the weight of the sheet feels excruciating."

This megagrief can last for hours or days, but a gout bout can vanish almost as swiftly as it comes, leaving you totally pain-free until the next episode. If you've had that experience, here's how to avoid a future round with the crystal attackers.

Lose weight, but not too quickly. The majority of gout patients are overweight—usually 15 to 30 percent over their ideal weights. The greater your girth, the higher your uric acid level. And the more uric acid, the more frequent and more intense the gout attacks. But lose weight gradually: A crash diet can actually raise uric acid levels.

Control your blood pressure. Gout patients with hypertension have twice as much to worry about. That's because some blood pressure medications boost uric acid levels, says Branton Lachman, Pharm.D., clinical assistant professor of phar-

FOODS TO AVOID

The best way gout patients can avoid a purine-packed flare-up is to avoid foods high in purine. Among the most loaded, containing from 100 to 1,000 milligrams per 3½-ounce serving:

Anchovies	Kidney	Poultry
Brains	Liver	Roast beef
Consommé	Meat extracts	Sardines
Gravies	Mincemeat	Sweetbreads
Heart	Mussels	
Herring	Pork roast	

The following foods should be limited to no more than one serving daily, since they contain 9 to 100 milligrams per 3½-ounce serving.

Asparagus	Luncheon meats	Peas (dry)
Beans (dry)	Mushrooms	Spinach
Lentils	Oatmeal	

macy at the University of Southern California School of Pharmacy in Los Angeles. His advice: Try to control your blood pressure naturally by decreasing sodium intake, exercising regularly, reducing excess weight and controlling stress.

Live without liver. Foods high in a substance called purine contribute to higher levels of uric acid. "You can't get away from purine, because it's in most foods," says Dr. Caldron. "But it's useful to avoid red meat, especially organ meats, some types of fish and even some dark green, leafy vegetables such as spinach."

Eschew the brew. Alcohol is a double whammy for those with gout, because it boosts the production of uric acid, says rheumatologist John G. Fort, M.D., clinical associate professor of medicine at Thomas Jefferson University Hospital in Philadelphia. Beer is particularly bad, because it has an even higher purine content than wine or other spirits.

But drink lots of water. You can help your kidneys flush excess uric acid from your system by going heavy on H_2O. (Besides, dehydration can trigger an attack.) "Brisk urinary output certainly may help," says Dr. Caldron. To accelerate "urinary output," Robert H. Davis, Ph.D., professor of physiology at the Pennsylvania College of Podiatric Medicine in Philadelphia, recommends no fewer than five glasses of water each day.

Reach for ibuprofen. It is the tremendous inflammation around an affected joint that causes the pain. So when you need a painkiller, says Jeffrey R. Lisse, M.D., an assistant professor of rheumatology at the University of Texas Medical School at Galveston, make sure it's one that can reduce inflammation—namely ibuprofen. Follow bottle directions. But if those dosages don't give relief, he says, consult your doctor before increasing them.

Avoid aspirin or acetaminophen. All pain relievers are not created equal. Aspirin can actually make gout worse by inhibiting excretion of uric acid, says Dr. Lisse. And acetaminophen doesn't have enough inflammation-fighting capability to do much good.

Give your sex life a kick. Urinating isn't the only way to get rid of uric acid. One study showed that, among men, frequent sexual activity reduces uric acid levels. The study suggests that more sex means less gout—for men, anyway.

Be sweet to your feet. Injure a big toe and you increase gout risk, say researchers. So wear shoes around the house to protect your feet from everyday accidents.

GUM PAIN

They say that pain is nature's way of ringing us up to tell us something's wrong. But when it comes to our gums, nature doesn't always use the hotline. More often, the message of gum pain seems to come via the old-time pony express: By the time we finally get the news, the situation at the point of origin is likely to have gone from bad to worse. So if your gums are hinting that something unusual is going on, it may be an understatement.

But *why* do gums hurt? "The causes could be either serious infections caused by bacteria or a situation where the skin on the gums has something wrong with it," says Kenneth Kornman, D.D.S., Ph.D., clinical professor and former chairman of the Department of Periodontics at the University of Texas Health Science Center at San Antonio. There are many infectious conditions that can cause pain. And every now and then, gum surfaces can be plagued with a maddening host of abrasions, burns, growths and lesions.

But all these problems have one thing in common: If they persist, they can really gum up your life, so don't take any chances when pain makes a rare cameo appearance. Head for the dentist's chair as soon as possible. Fast action now can save a lot of grief later.

And meanwhile, take these steps to find some relief.

Brush away gum pain. Removing bacteria with regular tooth care not only prevents gum disease, it can also provide some short-term pain relief, says Dr. Kornman. Proceed with gentle brushing (with a soft brush), flossing and warm-water rinsing. In addition, an over-the-counter rinse like Listerine, diluted or at full strength, may diminish some of the bacteria and ease some pain. (For some people, though, the alcohol content of a rinse may make pain worse. Discontinue using it if that happens.)

Don't rub. Massaging your gums may only cause further irritation, says Dr. Kornman.

Try a warm saltwater rinse. "Take a few swigs of warm salt water and swish it between your teeth and gums," advises Leslie Salkin, D.D.S., director of postgraduate periodontics and professor of periodontology at the Temple University School of Dentistry in Philadelphia. "It has a general soothing effect. If you have an abscess, the salts will help draw it out and drain it." He recommends one teaspoon of salt in a glass of lukewarm water. (Salt water is also your first line of defense for any gum burn, cut, abrasion or wound.)

Suppress the pain with an analgesic. Any over-the-counter medicine that reduces pain and inflammation could do wonders for your sore gums. It can also help reduce a fever if your pain is caused by an infection. "We're finding that in most cases of dental disease, it is inflammation that causes discomfort," says Samuel Low, D.D.S., associate professor and director of graduate periodontology at the University of Florida College of Dentistry in Gainesville. "Consequently we are recommending anti-inflammatory products such as ibuprofen [Advil]." Or you can take aspirin if you don't have adverse reactions to it (but children should avoid aspirin because of the risk of Reye's syndrome).

Don't put aspirin on your gum. "For some reason, many people have the idea that applying aspirin directly to the affected gum area is beneficial," says Kenneth H. Burrell, D.D.S., director of the American Dental Association's Council on Dental Therapeutics in Chicago. That couldn't be *farther* from the truth, he notes. "Unfortunately, the only thing that happens is that you create a chemical burn in the gum tissue. Don't ever try it."

Ice it down. For an all-natural anti-inflammatory, Dr. Low recommends ice. "It really works on swelling," he says, "and also serves as a local anesthetic to dull nerve endings." Apply an ice pack to your cheek or lip near the area of pain.

Moisten your mouth. Dr. Salkin recommends sucking on ice chips or a lemon drop if you are suffering from gum irritation due to dry mouth. That should be enough to replenish any missing saliva.

Use peroxide power. Many of the bacteria that cause gum pain cannot survive in oxygen, so some dentists recommend the use of everyday hydrogen peroxide, which you can pick up at any pharmacy and dilute. Dr. Low advises using a rinse of half water, half hydrogen peroxide.

Dab with baking soda. Another way to discourage bacteria is with household baking soda. Just make a paste of baking soda mixed with water and apply it gently on the gums, suggests Dr. Low. But be careful. Overzealous use can abrade gum tissue.

Numb that gum. If you have a burn, a cut, an ulceration or any problem on the skin of the gum, Dr. Kornman says the best thing you can do is apply one of the many over-the-counter gels or ointments that contain benzocaine. Its numbing action delivers instant relief. It also knocks out much of the pain associated with serious gum infections.

Anyone for tea? Some doctors suggest holding a wet tea bag against a gum abrasion or canker sore. Tea leaves contain tannic acid, an astringent that also has some pain-relieving power.

Say no to tobacco. "We see greater gum destruction in smokers," warns Dr. Salkin. He points out that smoking contributes to gum problems and can exacerbate any infectious or ulcerative conditions. Chewing tobacco is another gum irritant and can lead to a variety of gum cancers, according to Dr. Salkin. In addition, smoking often contributes to the onset of trench mouth and worsens the condition if you already have it.

HAY FEVER

There's no arguing that the thoughts of many knaves and maids turn to love when spring has sprung. But if you're one of those who gets hay fever in this festive season, then your libido isn't the only part of your body in overdrive.

Your nose may be stuffy or runny. Your eyes may itch and water. Your throat may feel irritated. You may even get hives when the bees leave theirs to do some pollinating.

Ah, spring . . . uh, better make that ahhh-chooo spring . . . but the truth is, this season has taken a bad rap from snifflers. Hay fever *isn't* solely a rite of spring; autumn brings its own share of misery. In the fall, when ragweed and other plants are blooming and spreading their windblown pollen everywhere, your respiratory system is one of the miserable landing sites.

And while a little congestion and sneezing may be a small price to pay to enjoy the wonders of Mom Nature's handiwork, here's how to get some wholesale relief for your sinuses *and* enjoy the Great Outdoors.

Make a routine of antihistamine. It's a common mistake: A hay fever sufferer takes one over-the-counter antihistamine, feels better and then waits until the symptoms are really bad before taking another one. But this can make you feel like you're on a roller coaster—feeling good one day and bad the next, says allergist William W. Storms, M.D., associate clinical professor of medicine at the University of Colorado School of Medicine in Denver. So if your doctor advises you to go the antihistamine route, it's important to take your medicine every day as a preventive during the allergy season.

Build up gradually. For maximum relief, take an antihistamine 30 minutes before going outdoors, suggests Gerald Klein, M.D., director of the Allergy and Immunology Medical Group in Vista, California. If one kind of antihistamine makes you drowsy, purchase a lower dose and take the lower dose just at bedtime for three days. (Antihistamines are formulated in different concentrations; check the package to compare doses.) During the next few days, gradually increase the dose and also begin taking one tablet in the morning, in addition to your nighttime tablet. "Dosing yourself gradually will help your body build up tolerance to the side effects, so you won't get so sleepy," says Dr. Klein. (He also suggests asking your doctor about nonsedating antihistamines, available by prescription.)

Don't be an early bird. Pollen counts tend to peak between 5:00 A.M. and 10:00 A.M., so limiting outdoor activity during the morning hours can help keep your allergies to a minimum. That means limiting exercise and other activities until mid- to late afternoon, when pollen is at its lowest, advises Dr. Klein. (You can also check prevailing winds and pollen counts in the newspaper, and they're mentioned in some radio and television weather forecasts.)

Go easy on the nasal sprays. Despite the temptation, don't use over-the-counter nasal sprays for longer than three days in a row. After that, they can actually increase congestion—and can even lead to addiction. "What happens with continued use is that the nose tissue becomes irritated and swollen and you feel even more stuffed up," explains Charles H. Banov, M.D., clinical professor of medicine and microbiology/immunology at the Medical University of South Carolina in Charleston and past president of the American College of Allergy and Immunology. "So you require more and more of the medicine for the tissue to shrink."

A safe, nonaddictive alternative for fighting nasal congestion is to inhale salt water, says Dr. Banov. Use one teaspoon of salt to one pint of water, plus a pinch of baking soda, and stir until both dissolve. Then place a few drops in a small spoon and sniff it up each nostril.

Run the air conditioner. Keep your house and car windows closed and your air conditioner on during spring, summer and fall months, advises H. James Wedner, M.D., chief of clinical allergy and immunology at Washington University School of Medicine in St. Louis. "If you don't want cooled air, at least flip on the fan setting. The fan will filter out the offending pollen." He also suggests, "During the pollen season, you should clean your air conditioner filter approximately once a month."

Use your clothes dryer. "Wind-dried clothes can become pollen catchers," says Dr. Klein. And when you wear them, you get a full dose. But drying clothes in a dryer, or hanging them inside to dry, will keep them pollen-free.

Lather your locks. After being outside for a long time during the day, wash your hair to avoid inhaling pollen that falls from your hair onto your pillow, suggests Robert Scanlon, M.D., clinical professor and director of the Allergy Clinic at Georgetown University Medical Center in Washington, D.C. If it's not possible to take a shower every evening, at least try to thoroughly wash your face, hands and eyes.

Watch out for melon. Having hay fever can make you more prone to food allergies. Researchers note that many people seem to have an allergic-like reaction after eating certain foods— what's called cross-reactivity. For instance, those allergic to ragweed often experience cross-reactive symptoms when they eat watermelon, cantaloupe or honeydew. Those with birch tree–pollen allergies sometimes react to cherries, apples, pears, peaches, carrots and potatoes. Herbal teas may also produce an adverse reaction in some people.

Ingestion of those foods does not produce hay fever. But it does bring on annoying symptoms such as "itching of the throat and swelling of the lips and tongue," says Robert Bush, M.D., chief of allergy at William S. Middleton Veterans Administration Hospital in Madison, Wisconsin, and professor of medicine at the University of Wisconsin–Madison. "If eating certain foods produces these or more severe symptoms such as breathing or swallowing problems, the best course is avoidance of the foods."

HEARING LOSS

When someone tells you there's a fast bat flying out of the barn and you think they're saying a fat cat is flying over the corn, you might as well face it: Your hearing is going. And it didn't just walk out the door today.

"The type of hearing loss experienced by most adults probably started when they were kids," says Robert E. Brummett, Ph.D., a pharmacologist at the Oregon Hearing Research Center in Portland. "Most people's hearing gets worse so slowly that they don't realize what's happening until they have severe hearing loss."

Most adults over age 60 do have *some* hearing loss. But any hearing problem can be greatly reduced by working with an audiologist or an otolaryngologist (ear, nose and throat doctor), according to Denise Wray, Ph.D., associate professor of speech and language pathology at the University of Akron. While hearing loss is usually irreversible, you owe it to yourself to take advantage of technology. "That means getting yourself outfitted with the best hearing aids and assistive listening devices possible," says Sam Trychin, Ph.D., director of a Coping with Hearing Loss Program at Gallaudet University in Washington, D.C. But whether or not you have a hearing aid, here are some hear-better strategies that will make everyone more audible.

Make some sound choices. "Whenever you walk into a room, make a quick appraisal of what might present problems," Dr. Trychin suggests. Reduce the background noise as much as possible by turning off the TV or radio when you have a conversation, adds Sharon A. Lesner, Ph.D., professor of audiology at the University of Akron. "And if the noise around you is out of your control, move to another room to talk," she suggests.

Dine away from din. "In a restaurant, position yourself away from the kitchen and away from the entrance," says Dr. Lesner. Ideally, choose a booth with a high back, so you can hear the person sitting across from you. Or sit with your back against a wall, so there's a "sounding board" behind you.

Look **to listen better**. You'll be able to understand more if you can see more. "Make sure light is on the face of the person you're trying to listen to. And if you wear glasses, make sure your vision is as good as possible," says Dr. Lesner. You don't have to be an expert lip-reader to pick up on visual signals that help people communicate. But you do hear better if you watch lip movement and expressions.

Speak up for yourself. "Be assertive about what you need speakers to do so that you can understand them," says Dr. Lesner. "For example, you might politely tell a person to slow down. Ask her to rephrase—not repeat—what she said. Or tell her what you believe she said and ask her if that is correct."

Block that clatter. Even if you already have hearing loss, you can further damage your hearing if you are in noisy situations. "Tie a pair of ear plugs or an earmuff-type hearing protector to any noisy equipment you might use," Dr. Brummett suggests. These personal "mufflers" will remind you to protect your ears.

Double the noise stoppers. "If you're going to be in a very noisy situation—using a power saw, for instance—wear both foam earplugs and earmuff-type protectors," Dr. Brummett suggests. The more protection, the better.

HEART PALPITATIONS

There's nothing like an off-beat ticker to scare the daylights out of you. Some irregularities in heartbeat are considered harmless and self-correcting. You may sense that your heart has skipped a beat, a condition known as ectopic (from the Greek *ektopos*, "misplaced") atrial heartbeat. Or your heart may suddenly speed up, a condition called tachycardia.

Sometimes this kind of arrhythmia passes quickly, with no serious effects. But—and this is a big but—only a doctor can say with certainty that your heart palpitations are nothing to worry about. "If you have any question about what you are experiencing, the safest thing is to have it checked out," says Jeremy Rushkin, M.D., director of the Cardiac Arrhythmia Service at Massachusetts General Hospital and associate professor of medicine at Harvard Medical School, both in Boston. That advice holds true whether you're young or old. (And even if other heart problems are ruled out during an exam, the doctor may want to prescribe medication specifically for arrhythmia.)

"People are often unaware of how they are setting themselves up for an arrhythmia problem," says Stephen Sinatra, M.D., chief of cardiology and director of medical education at Manchester Memorial Hospital in Manchester, Connecticut, and assistant clinical professor of medicine at the University of Connecticut School of Medicine in Farmington. "They need to address a number of things that could be contributing to their problem."

Here are some steps to consider.

If you smoke, stop. "Smoking is an extremely dangerous activity if you have cardiac arrhythmia," Dr. Rushkin says. "It can undo even the best of medical care."

Warm up and cool down. If you exercise, add at least ten minutes to the beginning and end of your routine to give your heart time to change pace gradually. And no 50-yard dashes to the bus stop or sudden sprints up the stairs, unless you've warmed up first with a few passes around the block.

"Sudden exercise is a very common trigger in people prone to arrhythmia," Dr. Rushkin says. Cooling down is equally important, especially if you've been running, cycling or doing other exercises that involve your legs, Dr. Rushkin says.

Save skydiving for another lifetime. If you've never had arrhythmia, chances are you won't develop it pursuing even the most daring of avocations. "But if you're prone to arrhythmia, we suggest you not put yourself into such stressful circumstances," Dr. Rushkin says. That goes for occupational stress, too. A firefighter or policeman may need to switch to a less hair-raising job.

Stick with noncompetitive sports. "I have the opportunity to take care of a number of competitive athletes with heart arrhythmias, and they tend to have problems only when they are in a competitive situation," says Dr. Rushkin. "The combination of competition and physical stress is a much more powerful trigger of arrhythmias than is either one alone, and that's not surprising."

Restrain yourself at all-you-can-eat buffets. Stuffing yourself to the gills—what doctors politely call metabolic overload—can bring on heart palpitations in those prone to them, Dr. Rushkin says. So eat lightly.

Go easy on alcohol. "Some people with arrhythmias are extremely sensitive to alcohol, and they usually know it—they sometimes get palpitations after just one drink," Dr. Rushkin says. "We advise them to be very cautious and moderate in their drinking. I prefer that they not drink at all."

Say no to joe. Coffee, tea, chocolate and certain drugs that contain caffeine, such as diet pills, can exacerbate arrhythmia problems in some people. "I recommend that people who have a history of arrhythmias should avoid caffeine as much as possible," says Dr. Rushkin.

Give your medicine chest the twice-over. Quite a few drugs can cause heartbeat problems, including those sometimes prescribed to correct arrhythmia. Culprits include digitalis, beta blockers, calcium channel blockers, all antiarrhythmic drugs, tricyclic antidepressants and cimetidine (Tagamet), a popular ulcer drug.

"A doctor can sometimes tell early on that a drug is going to cause problems, and that's why many of these drugs are started in the hospital," Dr. Rushkin says. "But some effects may occur later and may occur unexpectedly." Contact your doctor immediately if you think you're having a problem.

And be especially wary of decongestants. Even popular over-the-counter drugs can cause problems, says Dennis Miura, M.D., Ph.D., director of cardiac arrhymthias and electrophysiology at Albert Einstein College of Medicine of Yeshiva University in the Bronx. "Decongestants and asthma sprays that contain ephedrine or pseudoephedrine are the most common offenders," he says. They can cause a faster and somewhat more forceful heart rate and, in some circumstances, can cause or exacerbate serious arrhythmias. If you're already prone to arrhythmia problems, don't use these drugs without your doctor's okay.

Breathe calmly and fully. If you tend to hold your breath, as some people do when they're frightened, tense or straining in some physical activity, or if your breathing is shallow and rapid, you can upset your heart's natural rhythm, says Robert Fried, Ph.D., director of the Biofeedback Clinic at the Institute for Rational Emotive Therapy in New York City and author of *The Psychology and Physiology of Breathing in Behavioral Medicine.* So pay attention to your breathing. Allow yourself to exhale fully, then relax your belly and give your lungs time to fill before you exhale again.

Try the vagal maneuver. How fast your heart beats and how strongly it contracts are regulated by sympathetic nerves and parasympathetic nerves (or vagal nerves). When your heart pounds, the sympathetic network is dominant. (That's the system that basically tells your body to speed up.) What you want to do is switch control to the mellower parasympathetic network. If you stimulate a vagal nerve, you initiate a chemical process that affects your heart the same way that slamming on the brakes affects your car. One way to do this is to take a deep breath and bear down, as if you were having a bowel movement, says John O. Lawder, M.D., a family practitioner specializing in nutrition and preventive medicine in Torrance, California.

Roll with the punches. "I am convinced that stress can be a powerful factor in enhancing or increasing susceptibility to arrhythmia," Dr. Rushkin says. "I would certainly endorse any program or activity that reduces stress. People simply need to find what works best for them." Meditation, biofeedback, yoga, prayer, music—all can ease tension.

Fill up on fish. Preliminary studies from researchers in Australia suggest that omega-3 fatty acids from fish such as salmon and mackerel may help reduce arrhythmias. The researchers think these fats may alter the composition of heart muscle cells, making them less prone to rhythmic disturbances.

HIGH BLOOD PRESSURE

Poor diet, lack of exercise, heavy-duty weight training, even innocuous-sounding activities such as public speaking can make your blood pressure leap. But when your blood pressure goes up and stays up, there's cause for concern: Of all the risk factors for heart attack, high blood pressure remains the most accurate predictor of who will get cardiovascular disease after age 65.

Anyone with high blood pressure needs to be under a doctor's care—not only for regular monitoring but often for medication as well. The good news is that many of the 60 million Americans with high blood pressure can do something about it without drugs. If you're among them, your doctor has no doubt mentioned the importance of regular exercise, avoiding smoking, managing stress and changing your diet to put limits on alcohol, salt and fats. But here are some lesser-known factors that can take your blood pressure down a notch or two and significantly slash your risk of heart failure, stroke and kidney disease.

Munch on celery. Celery and its oil have been used in oriental folk medicine for centuries to treat high blood pressure and circulatory problems, and now the West may know why. University of Chicago researchers have found that a compound in the vegetable helps lower blood pressure by relaxing muscles lining the arteries. This allows the muscles that regulate blood pressure to dilate.

Best of all, it doesn't take much to reap the rewards. Eating the equivalent of four stalks a day can lower blood pressure in rats an average of 13 percent, reports William Elliott, M.D., Ph.D., assistant professor in the Department of Preventive Medicine at Rush–St. Luke's–Presbyterian Medical Center in Chicago.

And gobble down garlic. The reason isn't as well established, but garlic is another blood pressure buster. "We know that eating garlic can lower your blood pressure, but we're still trying to learn exactly why," says Yu-Yan Yeh, Ph.D., associate professor of nutrition at Pennsylvania State University in University Park and a leading researcher on the healing properties of garlic. "Eating as little as one clove a day—either raw or used in cooking—seems to have a beneficial effect."

Note: In animal studies, garlic has also been shown to lower cholesterol and triglycerides—other factors that have an impact on heart disease. And it doesn't matter whether you eat fresh garlic or take it in a capsule: In either form, it has the beneficial effect.

Pass the potassium, please. Increased levels of this mineral may be valuable in helping control high blood pressure. "The number of hypertensives who respond to potassium seems to depend on how long the studies are performed," says George Webb, Ph.D., a professor in the Department of Physics and Biophysics at the University of Vermont College of Medicine in Burlington. "In a two-week study, we find that maybe 30 percent get a reduction, but with an eight-week study, we might find that 70 percent get a reduction," he says.

Dr. Webb believes that the total amount of potassium you consume isn't as important as maintaining the correct sodium/potassium ratio in your diet. "We believe there's a clear benefit when you get three times as much potassium as sodium," he says. "If you're on a low-salt diet and getting 2 grams of sodium (2 grams of sodium equals 5 grams of table salt) per day, then you should get 6 grams of potassium."

How do you know if you're getting enough? Well, it's virtually impossible to devise a low-salt diet that's not high in potassium. "And it's hard to avoid potassium if you eat plenty of natural foods," says Dr. Webb. Potatoes, fresh fruit, and fish are loaded with it. To calculate ratios, however, you may need to consult the tables of a nutrition reference book.

Make the calcium connection. "Calcium seems to have a favorable effect on some people," says Roseann Lyle, Ph.D., an

HOME TREATMENT HELPER

Perhaps the best thing you can do for yourself once you've been diagnosed with high blood pressure is to invest in a home blood pressure monitor. A daily measurement of your blood pressure can indicate whether your medication and home remedies are actually working to lower your blood pressure.

But even if you notice an improvement, don't stop taking a doctor-prescribed medication unless you have your physician's approval, advises David Spodick, M.D., director of clinical cardiology at St. Vincent Hospital at the University of Massachusetts Medical School in Worcester. You'll be most likely to remember your medication if you establish a routine, such as taking it immediately before breakfast or right after you walk your dog each morning.

---

assistant professor of health promotion and education at Purdue University in West Lafayette, Indiana. But the search to discover exactly who will respond favorably to calcium continues.

"It seems that salt-sensitive hypertensives, who may be about half the people with high blood pressure, are the same ones who respond well to calcium," says Lawrence M. Resnick, M.D., assistant professor at The New York Hospital–Cornell University Medical Center in New York City. "So if salt is bad for you, calcium's good for you."

Get a pet. "We know that when people touch or pet their animals, there's almost always a small but significant drop in blood pressure," says Alan Beck, Sc.D., coauthor of *Between Pets and People* and professor of ecology at Purdue University School of Veterinary Medicine. "Even just *looking* at an animal, such as a fish in a tank, results in a consistent drop in blood pressure. Being around animals seems to put people at ease and help reduce their stress."

Speak softly. According to some studies, simply speaking loudly and rapidly can significantly raise your blood pressure during normal conversation. And if people do this while engaged in emotional exchanges, especially angry ones, their blood pressure can shoot up even higher, says Aron Siegman, Ph.D., professor of psychology and director of the Behavioral Medicine Program at the University of Maryland, Baltimore County, in Catonsville.

Chronic anger-produced elevations in blood pressure may be a serious risk factor for coronary heart disease, according to Dr. Siegman. "As people raise their voices, it increases their blood pressure, and as their blood pressure goes up, they tend to raise their voices further in an ever-increasing cycle that tends to turn anger into rage," he says. The good news is that speaking softly and slowly, even about the most anger-provoking events, totally eliminates the cardiovascular upheaval.

Don't lie around. Besides speaking softly, speak the truth. Lying has been found to boost blood pressure, because it requires more brain function. The more you lie, the more you add stress (and, hence, increase your blood pressure), says David Robertson, M.D., director of the Clinical Research Center at Vanderbilt University School of Medicine in Nashville.

Make your exercise aerobic, *not* isometric. While regular exercise is one of the best ways to lower blood pressure, it has to be the right kind. Isometric exercises in which you clench and hold, such as weight lifting, should be avoided, says David Spodick, M.D., director of clinical cardiology at St. Vincent Hospital at the University of Massachusetts Medical School in Worcester. That's because heavy weight lifting can cause blood pressure to temporarily skyrocket, especially if you hold your breath while lifting (as most people do).

INFLAMMATORY BOWEL DISEASE

Stan hung up the phone with a bang. "Just my luck," he groaned. "Everyone from work—heck, everyone in town—will be at the game, and I'm stuck at home with this again!" He yanked up his T-shirt and gave the ailing offender, which hung dejectedly over the top of his belt, a resounding slap. As if on cue, an angry growl rumbled to the surface.

Few things could keep Stan down when his beloved Buzzards played at home, but this stubborn little bug, which hit all too often lately, was a devil. It gave him gas, stomach cramps and diarrhea five times a day. That's why he nixed the game. Even with courtside seats, he might not reach the men's room in time. But missing the game—*this* game—was the last straw. "Monday," Stan promised himself, "I'm going to see the doctor."

And it's a good thing he did. It didn't take his doctor long to realize Stan's "little bug" wasn't a stomach flu. After analyzing a stool culture, he knew Stan didn't have an intestinal infection either. Now he was getting suspicious, so he asked Stan to come back the following week for a colonoscopy—a procedure that lets the doctor take a close look at the inside of the intestine. That Monday, Stan showed up at the hospital right on time. The procedure went without a hitch, and a half hour later, the doctor's suspicions were confirmed. Stan had inflammatory bowel disease. "IBD," his doctor called it.

IBD is an intestinal disorder thought to afflict up to two million Americans with pain, cramping and bowel movement irregularities. There are many diseases that can cause inflammation in the bowel, but when doctors talk about IBD, they're usually referring to Crohn's disease or ulcerative colitis.

"Ulcerative colitis only affects the colon, and its primary symptom, in the early stages, is bloody diarrhea," says gastroenterologist Samuel Meyers, M.D., a clinical professor of medicine at Mount Sinai School of Medicine in New York City. Crohn's disease, on the other hand, can affect any part of the digestive tract. Its primary symptoms are abdominal pain, diarrhea and weight loss.

If Crohn's disease and ulcerative colitis sound similar, well, they are. That's why doctors may refer to them simply as IBD. But IBD could also stand for "incredibly baffling disease." That's because doctors don't know how to cure it. They aren't even sure what causes it, although bacterial infections, a flawed immune system and hereditary links all are suspected. One study found that close relatives of people with IBD are ten times more likely to contract the disease than those without a family history of the disease.

INFLAMMATION FIGHTERS

The only thing that's really predictable about IBD is that it's *unpredictable*. Even though Stan has been plagued by his problems for about a year, he can still work all day on the dock, bowl a few games a month and, until recently, make it to all the Buzzards games. That's because most of the time he *feels* okay—his IBD is under control. Sure, he has diarrhea sometimes, but who doesn't? But when Stan's IBD flares up—usually for a few days every month—he feels bad, really bad. Then the gas, bloating and abdominal cramps hit with a vengeance. The only place he dares go is to the bathroom.

But Stan's reaction to IBD is not necessarily how *you* react to IBD. Everyone experiences IBD differently. For some people like Stan, the symptoms flare only occasionally; for others, the pain can be unrelenting. Some people get constipated; others have diarrhea so often they're afraid to leave the house. If the disease progresses long enough, people can suffer fever, dehydration and malnutrition. And although IBD strikes in dissimilar ways, Dr. Meyers warns, for all sufferers one thing is certain: It always comes back.

Drugs are the best way to quench the fire, says gastroenterologist Bernard M. Schuman, M.D., a professor of medicine at the Medical College of Georgia at Augusta. Unfortunately, there's no one perfect drug.

One of the drugs most commonly prescribed is sulfasalazine (Azulfidine). Containing both an antibacterial compound and a salicylate (a drug related to the active compound in aspirin), sulfasalazine helps ease painful flare-ups. Taken regularly, it can even help *prevent* flare-ups of ulcerative colitis and some stages of Crohn's disease. But sulfasalazine has its drawbacks: Nausea, headaches and allergic reactions are common side effects.

A related drug, 5-ASA (Rowasa), appears to relieve bowel inflammation without side effects. 5-ASA has been most effective when used rectally—in enemas—but there are also oral formulas (Dipentum), Dr. Schuman says. Researchers are trying to improve the oral formulas, he says.

But sulfasalazine and 5-ASA, although relatively safe, don't always work. That's why doctors often turn to the more powerful steroids.

Fast and efficient, steroids are the gold standard when it comes to beating inflammation. But prolonged use can lead to serious side effects, including high blood pressure and osteoporosis. Many doctors prescribe steroids only when less dangerous drugs won't do the trick.

A class of drugs called immunosuppressants can also help relieve the symptoms of IBD. For reasons that aren't yet clear, some people with IBD also have immune system–related diseases, such as arthritis. Doctors speculate that IBD, like rheumatoid arthritis, may be caused by a glitch in the immune system that, in effect, orders the body to attack itself.

However, the potential side effects of the immunosuppressants—pancreatitis, allergic reactions and even cancer—have made some doctors wary of using them.

KEEPING IBD AT BAY

Even though these drugs (and researchers are always looking for new ones) can help relieve the symptoms of IBD quickly, they work only when the disease is active—and you're already in pain. To help prevent the pain from getting started, doctors recommend the following.

Think small at mealtime. Because everyone reacts differently to different foods, it's tricky to recommend a one-food-fits-all diet, Dr. Schuman says. However, there is one rule worth following: Don't overeat. "People will usually do better if they eat frequent, small meals that are easily digested," Dr. Schuman says. In other words, a serving of rice might sit more easily than a Mexican buffet.

Know your fiber facts. Some doctors believe that people who don't eat enough dietary fiber may be at increased risk for IBD. Indeed, in countries where people routinely eat lots of fiber (and relatively little fat), IBD appears to be something of a rarity. But scientists aren't sure if it's the fiber or something else in the diet, or even the environment, that helps prevent IBD.

In fact, fiber can sometimes make IBD worse once symptoms of flare-up begin, Dr. Meyers says. When the symptoms are mild, however, fiber can help slow the flow of diarrhea by absorbing excess water from the gut. And for people whose symptoms lean more toward constipation, fiber can help move things along.

Empty the gas tank. Many people with IBD suffer from excessive gas and flatulence, Dr. Schuman says. The best way to prevent a gas attack is to avoid gas-producing foods—beans, for example, and broccoli and cauliflower. If milk and ice cream give you gas, you could be sensitive to lactose. Try avoiding dairy foods when your insides are aching. If you still have excessive gas no matter what you eat, drugs containing simethicone (Maalox is one example) may help, Dr. Schuman says.

Put it to bed. When things get bad, a little rest—make that a little bowel rest—can help, doctors say. The less strain you put on your insides, the less crampy they'll be. A diet of broths, purees and easy-to-digest foods helps relax the most irritable bowels. Just be sure you don't relax them too much. Many people with IBD simply don't get enough calories, protein, vitamins and minerals. You want to appease your bowels, not sacrifice a healthy diet.

Reach for relief. Keep over-the-counter antidiarrheal medicines on hand for those times when you are inconveniently hit with a bout of diarrhea (like on a day when you have to be in the office). Your doctor may prescribe Imodium or Lomotil— drugs that inhibit bowel contractions and slow the flow of diarrhea. In low doses, these drugs reduce the frequency of bowel movements without turning off the gut entirely, Dr. Schuman says.

Stop the stress. The less stress in your life, he says, the less the likelihood of recurrent flare-ups. If you have IBD, he recommends that you try to maintain as normal a lifestyle as possible. The more active you are, and the more satisfied you are with your life, the less you'll worry about your discomfort.

Friends can help. For some people, feeling good about themselves isn't all that easy. Some people, Dr. Schuman says, tend to suffer in silence. They shy away from talking about their problems. But people need to talk. That's why in many cities, people with IBD regularly get together. They form friendships, swap stories and talk about the different ways in which they cope with their symptoms. To learn about IBD support groups in your area, write to the Crohn's and Colitis Foundation of America, 444 Park Avenue South, New York, NY 10016.

Make peace with your insides. For many people, the worst part about IBD is that it rarely disappears altogether. Like bad weather, the pain, cramping and diarrhea always are on the horizon. It's important to be realistic about the disease, Dr. Schuman advises. "Your objective should be to reduce the discomfort to a level you can tolerate, even if that level may not be normal bowel function."

INTERMITTENT CLAUDICATION

Think of this condition as heart disease in your legs. The same circulatory problem that can restrict blood flow to your heart—atherosclerosis, or hardening of the arteries—is blocking the blood flow in your calves, thighs, feet or hips. The result: When you walk too far, you have severe pain in your legs, usually centered in the calves.

If you have intermittent claudication, you're a prime candidate for a heart attack or stroke, and you should be under a doctor's care. But there are several day-to-day things you can do to slow the progression of this peripheral circulatory problem—or perhaps even rid yourself of it completely.

Eat low-fat. "The oxygen in your blood isn't reaching your legs because of the plaques that line artery walls, causing atherosclerosis. And what causes those plaques is fat in your diet," says Arthur Jacknowitz, Pharm.D., professor and chairman of clinical pharmacy at West Virginia University School of Pharmacy in Morgantown. "So eliminating excess fat from your diet is essential for preventing or treating intermittent claudication."

Another benefit: A low-fat diet helps you lose weight, which is helpful for intermittent claudication and scores of other ailments.

Choose fish. Perhaps no food is better for those with intermittent claudication than fish—especially cold-water fish such as salmon, herring and mackerel. Besides being low in fat and high in nutrition, fish helps boost your levels of high-density lipoprotein (HDL), the so-called good cholesterol that scours fatty deposits from artery walls. "Tuna, sardines and some shellfish such as clams and mussels are also excellent," says Dr. Jacknowitz.

Take aspirin. Studies show that taking low-dose aspirin every other day helps reduce complications of peripheral vascular disease. Researchers believe that aspirin helps thin the blood, preventing circulation to the farthest parts of your body from getting worse.

Trash all tobacco. It's no mere coincidence that up to 90 percent of those with intermittent claudication are smokers. In fact, smoking is the single highest risk factor for peripheral vascular disease. Cigarette smoke increases the potential damage from the disease by substituting carbon monoxide for oxygen in the already oxygen-starved muscles of your legs. And nicotine constricts blood vessels, which further restricts blood flow. This can damage the arteries and may make blood cells more rigid, leading to blood clots. (Worst-case scenario: Clots can result in gangrene and make amputation necessary.)

"Unless you stop smoking, you won't receive any benefits from the other aspects of your treatment," warns Dr. Jacknowitz.

"Stopping smoking is the most important thing to do if you have intermittent claudication—period," notes Robert Ginsburg, M.D., director of the Unit for Cardiac Intervention at University Hospital in Denver and professor of medicine at the University of Colorado in Boulder.

Drink only now and then. Alcohol initially dilates blood vessels, which helps increase blood flow, but then has a rebound effect and constricts them (although not as much as smoking). An occasional beer or glass of wine is fine, but if you have intermittent claudication, it's not a good idea to drink regularly, experts say. In fact, people who drink chronically often develop intermittent claudication.

Hit the road. Although any type of regular exercise is good, the most helpful is walking. That's because walking improves blood flow to your legs and gives your circulatory system a boost where it needs it the most.

"Get out every day for at least an hour of walking exercise," suggests Jess R. Young, M.D., chairman of the Department of Vascular Medicine at the Cleveland Clinic Foundation in Cleveland.

Dr. Young says you don't have to walk that hour's worth all at once, "but for the walking to do any good, you have to bring on the discomfort of intermittent claudication." In other words, walk until you bring on the pain. But don't stop at the first sign of pain. "Wait until it gets moderately severe," says Dr. Young. "Then stop and rest a minute or two until it goes away, then start walking again."

Repeat that pain/walk cycle as often as you can during your 60 minutes of daily walking, he advises. And don't give up after a few weeks. Improvement will take several months.

Ban the heat. Because the blood flow in the legs is restricted, people who suffer from intermittent claudication often suffer from cold feet, too. If you're among them, don't warm your feet with a heating pad or hot water bottle.

"You need increased blood flow to help dissipate that heat," Dr. Young explains. "If the blood flow is limited, however, it can't get down to where you're putting the heat, and you'll burn the skin." Instead, warm your tootsies with loose wool stockings.

IRRITABLE BOWEL SYNDROME

Just as some people are the grumpy and irritable type, so, too, are some bowels. What exactly does it mean to have an irritable bowel? It means that certain foods and drinks and stressful events in your life—things that don't normally wreak havoc on other people—give you alternating bouts of diarrhea, constipation, and abdominal pain. Sometimes, you get all three at the same time.

Some doctors think that irritable bowel syndrome (also known as spastic colon) may be second only to the common cold as America's most widespread medical complaint. And your doctor now says that irritable bowel syndrome (IBS) is the source of *your* complaint. Well, rest assured that there are lots of things you can do to take the irritability out of your bowel.

Take the news in stride. "There's a very good connection between stress and an irritable bowel," says Douglas A. Drossman, M.D., a gastroenterologist and psychiatrist at the University of North Carolina at Chapel Hill School of Medicine. What you don't want to do is get stressed because you have an irritable bowel, and thereby create a "vicious cycle," he says. Especially during flare-ups of abdominal pain, it is important to "take a deep breath. Think about what's happening. Recognize that it's happened before and it will pass. Know that you're not going to die—because people don't die from an irritable bowel," he says.

Keep a stress diary. Persons with an irritable bowel have an intestinal system that overreacts to food, stress and hormonal changes. "Think of your irritable bowel as a built-in barometer, and use it to help you determine what things in your life are most stressful," says Dr. Drossman. If, for instance, you have stomach pain every time you talk to your boss, see it as a sign that you need to work on that relationship (perhaps by talking it over with your boss, a friend or family member, or a therapist).

GET RID OF GAS WITH BEANO

Beans, cabbage and carbohydrates from veggies can cause gas. And for someone with irritable bowel syndrome (IBS), eating a simple meal can lead to uncomfortable aftereffects.

But there is a way to have your chili and eat it, too. "An over-the-counter product called Beano does reduce the gas caused by many foods and certainly can help those with IBS," says gastroenterologist Stephen B. Hanauer, M.D., professor of medicine in the Section of Gastroenterology at the University of Chicago Medical Center. "The key is to look at all the things that might be causing your IBS symptoms. Then if you're going to eat these foods, put in a few drops of Beano before you eat to halt any potential problems."

To help narrow down your list of possible offenders, note that IBS sufferers often have problems with spicy foods such as chili; gas-producing vegetables such as broccoli, cabbage and cauliflower; all types of legumes; fatty foods, which are hard to digest; and even carbohydrates such as bread and pasta.

Get a juicer. Most store-bought juices contain high amounts of sorbitol—especially fortified apple, peach, pear and prune juices, says Arvey I. Rogers, M.D., chief of the Gastroenterology Section at the Veterans Administration Medical Center in Miami and professor of medicine at the University of Miami School of Medicine. Since fruit juices are an excellent source of nutrients, you can make your own—with reduced sorbitol content—by using a commercial juicer that can be bought at most department stores.

Don't be too sweet on sweets. Controlling your sweet tooth is one of the best ways to put the bite on IBS-triggered diarrhea. "You have to be careful with sugars if you have IBS, especially fructose and the artificial sweetener sorbitol," says Stephen

B. Hanauer, M.D., professor of medicine in the Section of Gastroenterology at the University of Chicago Medical Center. That's because sugars, which are not easily digested, are a leading cause of the runs. His advice: Avoid candy and gum, which contain these sweeteners, and read food labels on other products.

Bulk up. Eating a high-fiber diet—between 35 and 50 grams daily, compared with the average 11 grams most Americans eat—is perhaps the best way of taking the irritability out of your bowels. "Fiber increases stool production and reduces pressure in the intestines, which is good for both constipation and diarrhea," says Dr. Hanauer. "It also allows for more regular bowel movements."

Since increased fiber usually causes more gas and can temporarily worsen symptoms, the slow and steady route is strongly recommended. "I advise my patients to start with ½ cup of oat or wheat bran high-fiber cereal [or three tablespoons of pure bran] every day at breakfast. I suggest they have a green leaf salad with lunch and dinner and plenty of fresh fruits and vegetables throughout the day," advises Alex Aslan, M.D., a gastroenterologist and staff physician at North Bay Medical Center in Fairfield, California. "Continue to slowly add the bran over a six-week period until you have 1 to 1½ cups each morning, while having two salads and lots of fruits and vegetables." Adequate fluid intake is also very important.

Reconsider dairy products. One fluid you may do better without is milk. "A large number of people who say they have IBS are really lactose intolerant," says William J. Snape, Jr., M.D., a professor of medicine, chief of the Gastroenterology Unit, and director of the Inflammatory Bowel Disease Center at the Harbor-UCLA Medical Center in Torrance, California. It means your body has difficulty absorbing lactose, an enzyme found in milk. Your doctor can test you for lactose intolerance, or you can give up dairy products for a couple of days and see how you do. In either case, you may find this one dietary change can clear up all your problems.

Meditate. Even when you're not eating, controlling the stresses in your life is a key factor in controlling IBS. "Being under stress will definitely make IBS worse," says Dr. Hanauer. "And not being under stress can help." You may benefit from relaxation techniques such as meditation, self-hypnosis, biofeedback, regular exercise or even keeping a "stress diary" to determine what's causing you (and your bowels) grief.

But don't medicate. You won't help yourself by relying on medicines to control diarrhea, constipation or other gastrointestinal problems. "Laxatives and antidiarrhea medications should be used only on a short-term basis—if at all," says Dr. Hanauer. The exceptions: Natural psyllium-based laxatives such as Metamucil or Citrucel can be taken daily to boost your fiber, and they actually cause less gas than bran.

Give pain the "heat-ho." For the abdominal pain of IBS, nothing beats a heating pad. Turn it on low heat and rest it on the painful area. Another warm-up strategy: Take a warm bath, says Dr. Rogers.

Don't be a coffee achiever. Coffee and other caffeinated drinks play a significant role in IBS—and it's not a beneficial one. "For one thing, caffeine, even in very small amounts, stimulates motility. And that's bad news if you're prone to diarrhea," says Dr. Aslan. "Even if you're not, there's an unknown chemical in coffee that can cause cramping." His advice: Either cut back or cut out coffee and limit intake of tea, chocolate, cola and other caffeinated substances.

PHLEBITIS

I t's a pain in the leg—or both legs. That's how it begins, anyway. And when the pain doesn't go away, you probably want to pick up the phone and call the doctor.

Well, that's exactly the right thing to do, because anyone with the warning signs of phlebitis needs to find out as soon as possible which kind of phlebitis he or she has. And only a doctor can tell you that.

Phlebitis (the full name is *thrombophlebitis*) is an inflammation or blood clot in a vein, usually in the legs. There are two kinds. Deep-vein thrombophlebitis is the risky variety. It affects the veins that are deep beneath the skin (that explains the name), and it can be fatal if a blood clot dislodges from the vein and travels to the lungs. So doctors recommend immediate action if an exam turns up any warning signs of deep-vein phlebitis.

More often the problem is superficial thrombophlebitis, which means that you have some blockage in the superficial veins near the surface of the legs. Painful, yes—but not dangerous. Be ready to call the doctor again if you see any sign that it's getting worse. But in the meantime, there are many things you can do to ease the pain and reduce the worry associated with this problem.

The tips here should be used only by people who have been diagnosed with superficial phlebitis and are under a doctor's care. If that means you, here's what you can do to reduce your chances of another bout with pain, redness, tenderness and itching in your legs.

Take a load off. "Superficial phlebitis can be treated by elevating the leg and applying warm, moist heat," suggests Michael D. Dake, M.D., chief of cardiovascular and interventional radiology at Stanford University Hospital in Stanford, California. Keep legs elevated 6 to 12 inches above the level of the heart, and apply a heating pad to the affected area. In fact, it may help to keep your feet up all night long. You can elevate the foot of your bed several inches with wooden blocks.

MASSAGE CAN BE DANGEROUS

I f you have phlebitis, you might be tempted to "massage away" the pain when you have a flare-up. But that's not advisable unless you have explicit permission from your doctor, according to Robert Ginsburg, M.D., director of the Unit for Cardiovascular Intervention at the University Hospital in Denver and professor of medicine at the University of Colorado in Boulder.

Massage can be dangerous for people who have superficial or deep-vein phlebitis, because you could dislodge a blood clot and cause a stroke or heart attack. So don't try hands-on healing without your doctor's blessing.

Put the pressure on. Any kind of exercise, but especially walking, allows you to stay one step ahead of phlebitis. Muscular activity puts pressure on the veins, which helps empty them. Essentially, the walking motion helps prevent pooling of blood in the veins, according to Robert Ginsburg, M.D., director of the Unit for Cardiovascular Intervention at the University Hospital in Denver and professor of medicine at the University of Colorado in Boulder.

Pop some aspirin. Besides reducing pain and easing inflammation, aspirin has blood-thinning properties, so it may reduce phlebitis by preventing rapid clot formation. For best results, take aspirin before prolonged periods of bed rest or travel, which are the times when your circulation is most sluggish. And if you're phlebitis-prone, your doctor may recommend aspirin before you have any kind of surgery.

But don't down the Pill. "If you've had a history of phlebitis or blood clots, you definitely shouldn't use oral contraceptives," says Jess R. Young, M.D., chairman of the Department of Vascular Medicine at the Cleveland Clinic Foundation in

Cleveland. (The incidence of *deep-vein* thrombophlebitis in oral contraceptive users is estimated to be three to four times higher than in nonusers.)

Think of zinc. If itching is a problem, a dab of zinc oxide in the bothersome areas can bring relief, according to Dr. Young. Zinc oxide is sold in drugstores and doesn't require a prescription.

Sock it to yourself. Many phlebitis sufferers find that it helps to wear support stockings (the same kind used to treat varicose veins). The rule of thumb: If the stockings ease the discomfort, wear them. However, wearing support hose won't prevent a recurrence of phlebitis if you've had it before.

Ease your air travel. "On airplanes you tend to be confined to your seat a lot more than when traveling by car. So if you've had phlebitis, this is a case where you ought to put on your elastic stockings before boarding, then get out of your seat and walk up and down the aisle every half-hour or so after taking off," advises Dr. Young.

And don't smoke. Another no-no is cigarettes, which can also cause recurring phlebitis in a more complicated circulatory condition called Buerger's disease.

PNEUMONIA

Richard Levine of Albuquerque eats well, sleeps well and looks like a weight lifter—the rewards for spending thousands of hard, hot days making bricks at one of the largest adobe-brick manufacturing plants in the Southwest. But despite nearly 60 years of robust good health, Richard has two weak points: his lungs.

"The first time I had pneumonia, I was a student at Berkeley in 1968," Richard remembers. "My chest hurt like crazy, and I couldn't breathe—it was terrible. When I went to the doctor, he listened to my lungs and slapped me into bed in the hospital for a week. I just couldn't move." Richard's second bout with pneumonia—and another week in the hospital—came ten years later. After the third time, he was fed up. He finally took his doctor's advice and stopped smoking. "You know, I haven't had pneumonia since," he says.

IT GETS YOU WHEN YOU'RE DOWN

Actually, it's not cigarettes that cause pneumonia but viruses and bacteria that move into your lungs and bronchi, causing infection, inflammation and congestion. Ironically, the germs that often cause pneumonia—*Streptococcus pneumoniae*, for example—normally live in your throat and airways, and they even dip into your lungs without causing trouble. It's usually when your guard is down—after years of smoking and drinking, for example, or when you've been sick with another illness—that your lungs become vulnerable to these everyday bugs, says Steven W. Stogner, M.D., a fellow in the Division of Pulmonary and Critical Care Medicine at Louisiana State University School of Medicine at Shreveport. "Any illness, especially that of the lung, can predispose you to pneumonia caused by an organism that would not otherwise be virulent," he says.

When it's mild, pneumonia can be mistaken for a cold, Dr. Stogner says. In more serious cases, it can put you to bed for days with wracking coughs, burning fever and teeth-chattering, bone-rattling chills. In fact, pneumonia ranks sixth among death-causing diseases, killing more than 40,000 Americans every year. This is because pneumonia often strikes people whose systems are already weakened by other underlying health problems, like heart disease, asthma or emphysema. "If you think you have pneumonia, you need to see a doctor," Dr. Stogner warns. "People can die from pneumonia."

Since pneumonia tends to strike when your natural resistance isn't up to snuff, the best way to prevent it is to stay in shape.

KEEPING IT AT BAY

Of course, no one is healthy all of the time, and it's impossible to avoid entirely the multitudes of pneumonia-causing germs (a few of which are nasty enough to get you even if you're in the best of health). But you can keep your defenses in fighting form and greatly reduce your chances of getting pneumonia. For starters:

Encourage coughs. "One of the risk factors for pneumonia is being unable to properly clear secretions from the airways," Dr. Stogner says. People who smoke or who have frequent colds or other respiratory tract infections will often harbor large amounts of mucus in their lungs and airways, he explains. Bacteria love phlegm. And the more bacteria you have in your airways, the greater your chances for getting pneumonia. In other words, those productive coughs—those that bring up phlegm—really are protective coughs.

Keep your distance. Some pneumonias are contagious while others are not, but catching a lungful of anyone else's germs is pushing your luck. If you're in the sickroom with someone with the disease, try to keep a few feet between you and whatever it is they're blowing, sneezing or coughing. Frequently washing your hands is added insurance, Dr. Stogner adds.

Snuff the cigarettes. Cigarette smoke essentially paralyzes the hairlike projections in your airways, called cilia, that help expel mucus and other secretions. If the cilia aren't working, the mucus—and hordes of bacteria—stay inside.

Fill up on fluids. Pneumonia's hot fevers will dry you out like the desert sun. You need to drink plenty of fluids—about six to eight glasses a day—to avoid dehydration.

Thin your phlegm. You already know how important it is to clear mucus from your lungs and airways. But because pneumonia often is accompanied by pleurisy, the slightest cough can be terribly painful. One possible solution to discuss with your doctor is to take over-the-counter drugs called expectorants. Essentially, these make your coughs more productive with less effort, Dr. Stogner says.

Lie on your side. By supporting, or splinting, your rib cage, this position should make coughing and breathing somewhat less painful.

Take some aspirin. Not only can aspirin help relieve your aches and pains, it will help cool your fever as well. Check with your physician about whether you should use aspirin or a substitute such as acetaminophen.

Get plenty of rest. Your lungs have been through the wringer, and they need time to recover, Dr. Stogner says. This isn't the time to overexert yourself. A gradual increase in daily activities is suggested.

PROSTATE PROBLEMS

Forget about those yearnings for red convertibles. The *real* midlife crisis occurs in a man's prostate, the gland that adds fluid to semen so that he can ejaculate. Four of every five men over age 50 develop an enlarged prostate—or, more specifically, a condition called benign prostatic hyperplasia (BPH). One-fourth to one-third of them will experience BPH's uncomfortable and potentially dangerous symptoms.

"BPH causes no pain, but it does make urination more difficult," says Stephen Rous, M.D., professor of surgery at Dartmouth Medical School and a urologist at Dartmouth-Hitchcock Medical Center in Lebanon, New Hampshire. Because the prostate surrounds the urethra, the tube that carries urine from the bladder, when it enlarges it restricts urine flow. This results in a need to urinate more frequently, often with increased difficulty getting started.

Surgery to remove the prostate is one alternative, and there are several medications—some of which take months to work—that can reduce an enlarged prostate and improve urination. But for tried-and-true *home* treatments, here's what the experts recommend.

Cut the caffeine. "Caffeine in any form—coffee, tea, chocolate or soft drinks—tends to tighten the bladder neck and make it more difficult to pass urine," says urologist Durwood Neal, Jr., M.D., associate professor of surgery, urology, microbiology and internal medicine at the University of Texas Medical Branch at Galveston. "Some of the prostate is made up of smooth muscle, and anything that causes that muscle to constrict will make urination more difficult. Caffeine does this quite a bit."

And banish booze. Alcohol also tightens the bladder neck to hamper urination. And since it's a diuretic, it increases the amount of urine that builds up inside the bladder, adds Dr. Neal. "Drinking alcohol also makes the bladder operate a lot less efficiently. And the more you drink, the more problems you'll likely have."

Give a cold shoulder to cold medicines. Antihistamines and decongestants can cause even more harm to some men. In fact, taking large doses of cold medications occasionally leads to urinary retention—a potentially life-threatening condition in which you completely stop urinating. "Decongestants cause the muscle at the bladder neck to constrict, restricting the flow of urine," says Peter Nieh, M.D., a urologist at the Lahey Clinic Medical Center in Burlington, Massachusetts. "And antihistamines simply paralyze the bladder."

If you have allergies as well as prostate problems, Dr. Nieh suggests you speak to your doctor about prescribing astemizole (Hismanal) or terfenadine (Seldane), two medications that have no antihistamines. If you must buy over-the-counter medication, take half the suggested dose. If no problem ensues, move to the full recommended dosage.

Be wary of spicy foods. Spicy and acidic foods bother some men with enlarged prostates, says Dr. Neal. "If you notice more problems after eating salsa, chili or other spicy or acidic foods, then you're among those men—and you should avoid that cuisine."

Manage your stress. Perhaps the most underrated trigger is unmanaged stress. "Stress plays a major role in prostate-related discomfort, because the bladder neck and prostate are both very rich with nerves that respond to adrenal hormones," says Dr. Neal. "When you're under stress, there are more of those hormones floating around—causing more difficulty in urinating."

Stress also triggers the release of adrenaline in your body, prompting a fight-or-flight response. "Just as it's impossible to get an erection during the fight-or-flight response, it can make urination difficult, too," Dr. Neal adds.

Get more amour. One way urologists help ease urination problems is to massage the prostate. For men with mild to moderate voiding difficulties, an alternative may simply be to have more sex. "Many men notice that the more they ejaculate, the easier it is to urinate," says Dr. Rous. That's because ejaculation helps empty the prostate of secretions that may hamper urination.

Empty your bladder before heading for bed. "Many men get the urge to urinate in the middle of the night, and it can be a real problem," says Dr. Neal. "But if you limit your intake of beverages after 6:00 P.M. and make sure you urinate before going to sleep, you can eliminate much of this problem."

Flee south in the winter. If at all possible, spend winters somewhere in the Sunbelt. "In the urology trade, we usually say that summer is the season to pass kidney stones and winter is the time for urinary problems. I'm not exactly sure why, but people have more trouble urinating and are most likely to go into urinary retention during cold weather. Perhaps this is due to an increase in upper respiratory infections, which many men treat with over-the-counter antihistamines and decongestants. These further aggravate BPH," says Harold Fuselier, M.D., chairman of urology at Ochsner Medical Institutions in New Orleans. "Since an enlarged prostate already makes urinating more difficult, you'll do much better in a warm climate during cold weather."

PSORIASIS

I f there ever was a medical condition that could convince Sherlock Holmes to get out of the business, it's psoriasis. The clues are obvious—after all, it's hard *not* to notice that maddening itch, the inflammation and those bothersome silvery scales that usually occur on the elbows, knees, trunk and scalp. But when it comes to finding its cause or cure, that's even more of a mystery than Watson's first name.

What is known about psoriasis is that it causes skin cells to go hyper. A normal skin cell takes about a month to mature, but in those with psoriasis, this process takes only three or four days. These skin cells are poorly developed, and they can't shed fast enough. Instead, they pile up—forming raised, scaly "plaques" that itch and leave skin below red and inflamed.

But instead of the proverbial heartbreak, there is reason to take heart. While there's no cure as yet, you can *control* psoriasis and lessen its impact on your life. Your doctor has probably told you about tar shampoos and ultraviolet light treatments, but here are some other ways to keep those plaques from giving you flak.

Look for lactic. All of our experts agree that the most important step in controlling psoriasis is to keep skin well moisturized. "A big problem with psoriasis is scale buildup, and moisturizers are extremely effective at preventing this," says Nicholas J. Lowe, M.D., clinical professor of dermatology at the University of California, Los Angeles, School of Medicine and director of the Skin Research Foundation of California in Santa Monica. "Plain petroleum jelly is a very effective moisturizer. But if you're buying a commercial moisturizer, those that contain lactic acid, such as LactiCare, seem to work better. Also, Eucerin cream works well as a moisturizer for those with psoriasis."

Moisturize after bathing. To get the most from your moisturizer, "apply it within three minutes after leaving the shower or bathtub," advises Glennis McNeal, public information director at the National Psoriasis Foundation headquarters in

Portland, Oregon. "We recommend that you pat yourself dry and apply the moisturizer liberally all over your body—*not* just on plaques. That's because even 'clear' skin in people with psoriasis is drier than in people who don't have psoriasis. It's thought that little cracks on dry skin might encourage more psoriasis."

Soak up the sun. Many psoriasis patients are prescribed a specific regimen of ultraviolet light treatments. Getting artificial sunlight from a special lamp or tanning booth can help. An easier and less expensive method is simply to hit the Great Outdoors. "We know that exposure to sunlight is extremely helpful for treating psoriasis," says David Kalin, M.D., a family practitioner in Largo, Florida. A moderate amount of sunlight enhances the production of vitamin D, which may be effective in controlling psoriasis.

But don't soak up the booze. Doctors are still trying to find out for sure why alcohol exacerbates psoriasis. They suspect that alcohol increases activity of a certain kind of white blood cell that's found in psoriasis patients but not in other people. (But it's also possible that drinkers are just more highly stressed—and therefore more prone to psoriasis.)

"Alcohol is a definite problem," says Stephen M. Purcell, D.O., chairman of the Department of Dermatology at Philadelphia College of Osteopathic Medicine and assistant clinical professor at Hahnemann University School of Medicine in Philadelphia. "It's best to *not* drink at all if you have psoriasis."

Spice up your bath. Bathing is often a catch-22 for those with psoriasis. That's because soaking in warm water helps soften psoriasis plaques, but it sometimes dries skin and worsens itching. "One way to get the benefits of a bath without the dryness is to add a couple of capfuls of vegetable oil to your bath," says McNeal. "The best way to do it is to get in the tub first, so your body soaks up the water, and then add the oil." Another alternative suggested by McNeal: Mix two teaspoons of olive oil in a large glass of milk and add that to your bath.

Be extra careful stepping out of the tub, since oils can make surfaces very slippery. (Be sure to scrub the tub afterward.)

Head to the kitchen to soothe that itchin'. To soothe itching caused by dry skin and psoriasis, dissolve ⅓ cup of baking soda in a gallon of water. Soak a washcloth in the solution, wring it out and then apply it to the itchy area. Or add a cup of apple cider vinegar to the water and apply that to the skin.

Cover the cracks with cow cream. If your skin is cracked because of psoriasis—which can cause itching and more plaques—do what dairymen do. "They found that Bag Balm, a product originally used to relieve cracking in cow udders, worked just as well on their cracked hands," says McNeal. "Then people with psoriasis found it worked great on their dry or cracked skin." Bag Balm is available at most feed stores; some drugstores may be able to order it.

Use tar without feathers. Over-the-counter coal tar preparations are weaker than the prescription versions but can be effective in mild psoriasis, says Laurence Miller, M.D., an adviser to the National Psoriasis Foundation and the National Institutes of Health. You can apply the tar directly to the plaques or immerse yourself in tar bath oil and treat your scalp with tar shampoo.

Since even the OTC tars can stain and smell, they're usually washed off after a certain amount of time, but some kinds can be left on the skin to enhance the effect of sunlight or UVB treatments. "Tar makes you more sensitive to the sun, so be careful," warns Dr. Miller.

He notes that some new tar products "have been made a little more elegant and cosmetically acceptable in gel form. They don't smell like tar pits, and they can be used daily and wash off easily." He gives these precautions: "If any tar product causes burning or irritation, stop using it. And tar should never be used on raw, open skin."

Take care of mind and body. Stress is a known trigger of psoriasis, so managing your mental state—through exercise, relaxation techniques or whatever mellows you out—is one way to keep your condition under control.

Watch what you eat. "Although there are no specific links that have been proven, it appears a diet high in oily fish—such as tuna, mackerel, sardines and salmon—helps reduce the itching and inflammation of psoriasis," says Dr. Lowe.

Avoid certain foods. "Some anecdotal reports suggest patients do better when they reduce or eliminate tomatoes and tomato-based dishes—possibly because of their high acidity levels," says Dr. Kalin. "Also, some of my patients with psoriasis have noticed a decrease in plaques by avoiding or limiting their intake of pork products and other fatty meats as well as caffeine."

Go electric. If you have plaques on your face, neck, legs or other areas that require shaving, use an electric razor instead of a blade. "An electric razor won't cut skin as easily, and every time you cut yourself, you risk new lesions," says dermatologist John F. Romano, M.D., clinical assistant professor of medicine at The New York Hospital–Cornell Medical Center in New York City.

RAYNAUD'S SYNDROME

You know Raynaud's syndrome all too well. You open a refrigerator door and your hands chill out in nothing flat. Or you notice changes in your fingers when you're punching away at your keyboard.

Suddenly the blood vessels to your fingers constrict. (Sometimes your toes are affected, too.) What you get at first is a spasm. Blood flow slows to the affected area, and that lack of oxygenated blood causes it to pale, maybe even take on a bluish tinge. Sometimes you experience a sensation of numbness from the lack of blood. Your fingers turn red again when the blood returns. In advanced stages of Raynaud's, poor blood supply can weaken the fingers and damage your sense of touch.

Cold isn't the only culprit. This odd but common affliction can result from injury to the blood vessels from the vibrations of powerful equipment like chain saws and pneumatic drills and from hypersensitivity to drugs that affect the blood vessels, or from disorders of the connective tissue. Other causes include nerve disorders.

How can you protect yourself from Raynaud's syndrome? Here's what our experts advise.

Condition yourself to overcome chills. Train your hands to heat up in the cold by adapting this technique that U.S. Army researchers in Alaska devised.

Choose a room that's a comfortable temperature and place your hands in a container of warm water for 3 to 5 minutes. Then go into a freezing room and again dip your hands in warm water for 10 minutes. The cold environment would normally make your peripheral blood vessels constrict, but instead, the sensation of the warm water makes them open. Repeatedly training the blood vessels to open despite the cold eventually enables you to counter the constriction reflex even without the warm water.

In the army experiments, this procedure was repeated every

other day for three to six times on 150 test people. After 54 treatments, the results were impressive. Their hands were 7 degrees warmer in the cold than before.

"People are training on the rooftops in New York City, in freezer lockers, in grocery stores, and in hospitals and hotels," says Murray Hamlet, director of the army's cold research program.

Twirl your arms to generate heat. You can actually force your hands to warm up through a simple exercise that Donald McIntyre, M.D., a dermatologist in Rutland, Vermont, devised. Pretend you're a softball pitcher. Swing your arm downward behind your body and then upward in front of you at about 80 twirls per minute. (This isn't as fast as it sounds; give it a try.)

The windmill effect, which Dr. McIntyre modeled after a skier's warm-up exercise, forces blood to the fingers through both gravitational and centrifugal force. This warm-up works well for chilled hands no matter what the cause is.

Eat iron-rich foods. Lack of iron may alter your thyroid metabolism, which regulates body heat. That's what researchers at the USDA Human Nutrition Research Center in Grand Forks, North Dakota, suspect. They measured the effects of dietary iron on six healthy women when they entered a cold chamber. When the women took only ⅓ of the recommended amount of iron for 80 days, they lost 29 percent more body heat than when they were on an iron-replete diet for 114 days.

Iron-rich foods include poultry, fish, lean red meat, lentils and leafy green vegetables. Orange juice is okay too, since it increases the body's ability to absorb iron.

Choose fabrics that wick away perspiration. Perspiration is an even bigger cause of cold hands and feet than temperature. Sweat is the body's air conditioner, and your body's air conditioner can operate in cold weather if you're not careful. The hands and feet are especially susceptible because the palms and heels (along with the armpits) have the largest number of sweat glands in the body. That's why the heavy woolen socks and fleece-lined boots you bought to keep your feet warm may instead make them sweaty and chilly.

Wear cotton-blend socks rather than pure cotton socks. You want to wear socks that wick moisture away from your feet and insulate them. All-cotton socks can soak up your perspiration and chill your feet. Those made of Orlon and cotton are a better choice.

Make sure garments are loose. None of your garments should pinch. Tight-fitting clothes, whether they are nylons, garter belts, jeans, or shoes, can cut off circulation and eliminate insulating air pockets.

Dress in layers. If you're stepping out into the cold, the best warming measure you can take is to dress in layers. This helps trap heat and allows you to peel off clothes as the temperature changes. Your inner layer should consist of one of the new synthetic fabrics, like polypropylene, which wicks perspiration away from your skin. Silk or wool blends also are acceptable. The next layer should insulate you by trapping your body heat. A wool shirt is one of your best options.

Waterproof your body. Choose a breathable, waterproof jacket or windbreaker. Gore-Tex shoes and boots are the best choice for keeping your feet warm and dry.

Wear a hat. Another good piece of clothing you can wear to warm your hands and feet is a hat. Your head is the greatest site of body heat loss. The blood vessels in your head are controlled by cardiac output and won't constrict like those in your hands and feet.

If you want to keep your hands and feet warm, says John Abruzzo, M.D., director of the Division of Rheumatology and a professor of medicine at Thomas Jefferson University in Philadelphia, it's as important to wear a hat as it is to wear gloves and socks.

Wear mittens. Mittens keep you warmer than gloves because they trap your whole hand's heat.

Try foot powder. Clothes aren't the only way to keep dry.
"Absorbent foot powders are excellent for helping keep feet dry,"
says Marc A. Brenner, D.P.M., a private practitioner in Glendale,
New York, and past president of the American Society of Podiatric
Dermatology. But he cautions people with severe cold feet problems caused by diabetes and peripheral vascular disease to use a
shaker can rather than an aerosol spray, since the mist from the
spray can actually freeze your feet.

Don't smoke. Smokers set themselves up for cold hands
and feet whenever they light up. Cigarette smoke cools you in two
ways. It helps form plaque in your arteries and, more immediately,
nicotine causes vasospasms that narrow the small blood vessels.
  These effects can be especially hard on people with Raynaud's.
"Raynaud's patients are sensitive even to other people's smoke,"
says Frederick A. Reichle, M.D., chief of vascular surgery at Presbyterian University of Pennsylvania Medical Center.

Chill out to warm up. Staying cool and calm may help
some people stay warm. Why? Stress creates the same reaction in
the body as cold. It's the fight-or-flight phenomenon. Blood is
pulled from the hands and feet to the brain and internal organs to
enable you to think and react more quickly.
  Calming techniques abound. Some, like progressive relaxation—in which you systematically tense, then relax the muscles
from your forehead to your hands and toes—can be practiced at
any time, in any place.

Pass on the coffee. Coffee and other caffeinated products
constrict blood vessels. The last thing you want when you have
Raynaud's syndrome is to interfere with your circulation.

Avoid alcohol. Don't be misled by the lure of a hot toddy,
either. Alcohol will temporarily warm up your hands and feet but

its detrimental effects outweigh its benefits as a hand and foot warmer.

Alcohol increases blood flow to the skin, giving you the immediate perception of warmth. But that heat is soon lost to the air, reducing your core body temperature. In other words, alcohol actually makes you colder. The danger comes from drinking an immodest amount and being subjected to unexpected cold for an extended period, which can lead to severe problems like frostbite.

Try mental heat. Perhaps the best way to beat Raynaud's is with your mind, says Robert R. Freedman, Ph.D., a Raynaud's expert and professor of psychiatry at Wayne State University Medical School in Detroit. Studies have shown that people who learn biofeedback can, with their minds, direct warming blood to their fingers—regardless of the temperature outside.

In training sessions at Wayne State, volunteers with Raynaud's were asked to monitor their finger temperatures while listening to a tone. When their temperatures changed, so did the pitch of the tone. Within a few sessions, Dr. Freedman says, they learned to raise their finger temperatures at will. "In every study we've done, the success rate has been 80 percent or better," he says.

Ask your doctor about finding a qualified biofeedback instructor in your area.

SEASONAL AFFECTIVE DISORDER

'Tis the month after Christmas, the goodies long gone.
But you're still overeating—what could be wrong?
You're depressed and blue and feeling real sick
And sporting a waistline like that of St. Nick.
All winter long, the story's the same:
Too little cheer, too much mental pain.
Can't figure why you can't get it together?
A winter's surprise: It could be the weather!

Okay, so it's not the lyrics of Clement Moore, but if you identify with that . . . ahem, *poem*, you've got something in common with one in five Americans—seasonal affective disorder (SAD).

For most people, the old "winter blues" simply mean that we feel a little run-down and melancholy in the season when we *should* be jolly. But for those who experience SAD at its most extreme, the blues hit harder than a flat note on a slide trombone. "We're talking about a condition that may compromise your life so seriously that you can't work or cope with your family, something that leaves you so lethargic that you can barely get out of bed," says George Brainard, Ph.D., associate professor of neurology and pharmacology at Jefferson Medical College of Thomas Jefferson University in Philadelphia and a leading researcher on the benefits of light therapy for SAD.

Symptoms of SAD may include a tendency to overeat, oversleep and even become disinterested in sex. But it doesn't have to get that far. Here's what to do to beat a major case of the blues.

Go with the glow. Although the *best* treatment for SAD is daily light therapy using a specially designed "light box," exposure to *any* type of bright light may help some people. "Flooding the room with bright, but not harsh, light actually helps some people," says Maria Simonson, Ph.D., Sc.D., professor emeritus

LIGHTEN UP YOUR MOOD

A surefire way to lighten up winter depression caused by seasonal affective disorder (SAD) is to undergo at-home therapy with a special lighting fixture. The most common type is known as a light box. This is a square fixture, usually a little larger than a briefcase, that stands upright on a desk or table. Other devices for treating SAD are configured as workstations, head-mounted visors or dawn simulators. Prices range from $200 to $500.

What's so special about a light box? "It's not so much that there's a magic bulb that works," says SAD light therapy researcher George Brainard, Ph.D., associate professor of neurology and pharmacology at Jefferson Medical College of Thomas Jefferson University in Philadelphia. "What's more important is the *dosage* emitted and the fact that it's emitted at *eye level.*"

The dosage is about five to ten times that of normal indoor lighting, and according to Dr. Brainard, you have to *look* repeatedly at the light; just having it fall on your skin isn't enough.

"The general prescription is two hours a day at 2,500 lux—a unit of light intensity," according to Dr. Brainard. He recommends that you set the light box in a position so that you can glance for a few seconds directly into the light. Glance at the light box about once a minute over the two hours. "Alternatively, some people use a 10,000-lux box for 30 minutes a day," says Dr. Brainard.

But before you plunk down your money, one last piece of advice: "First see a qualified physician or therapist and make sure you are diagnosed with SAD," says Dr. Brainard. "These lights won't work if you're just depressed; they'll only work if you have SAD." Your health professional can also advise you about reputable mail-order companies that sell light boxes.

and director of the Health, Weight and Stress Program at Johns Hopkins Medical Institutions in Baltimore. A word of caution: *Staring* into bright light emitted from lamps and overhead fixtures may harm your eyes, so don't stare at a bulb as a substitute for the light box.

Head for the Great Outdoors. The days are shorter in the winter, but you can still take advantage of what little sunlight there is. "*Any* exposure to sunlight will help," says Henry Lahmeyer, M.D., professor of psychiatry and behavioral sciences at Northwestern University Medical School and co-director of the Sleep Program at Northwestern Memorial Hospital, both in Chicago. "You should try to spend about an hour outdoors every day—even on days when it's not particularly bright and sunny."

Stroll in the dawn. "Research in Switzerland found that SAD patients who took an outdoor, 30-minute walk at sunrise showed a lot of improvement," says Dr. Brainard. "We're not sure whether it's the exercise, the sunlight or even the cold that invigorates them, but whatever it is, it seems to help."

Use your yoga. "Our research seems to indicate that some of the specific meditations in yoga may act on the pineal gland [which controls circadian and seasonal rhythms]," says Eric Leskowitz, M.D., a psychiatrist and SAD researcher at Spaulding Rehabilitation Hospital in Boston. "Yoga also provides a general energizing effect and offers great stress release. I think practicing yoga is a great way to start off the day if you have SAD."

Take milk for all it's worth. A form of vitamin D called soltriol that's found in milk may help keep us in sync with the sun, according to the theory based on a study by Walter E. Stumpf, M.D., Ph.D., a researcher at the University of North Carolina in Chapel Hill. The theory is that soltriol may trigger the release of "stimulating" hormones that keep our body clocks on track.

SLEEP APNEA

When it comes to comedy, whether it's Dagwood Bumstead's sofa antics or the Three Stooges and their sleeping sound effects, snoring has always given us a good laugh—and the louder the snarfing, gurgling and harrumphing, the louder our yuks.

But shake-the-walls snoring could be a sign of a potentially life-threatening condition called sleep apnea, in which the throat relaxes and closes during sleep. Sleep apnea affects nearly one of every ten Americans—primarily middle-aged to older men who are usually overweight.

"The difference between regular snoring and sleep apnea is that with sleep apnea, you actually *stop* breathing, anywhere from ten seconds up to three minutes," says Peter Hauri, Ph.D., co-director of the Mayo Clinic Sleep Disorders Center in Rochester, Minnesota. "And these stoppages are frequent—a minimum of at least 15 per hour. Usually the person stops breathing for 30 or 40 seconds and then gasps for air [making the snoring sound] and resumes breathing. For your bed partner, it can be most terrifying." And it could be dangerous as well—since people with sleep apnea have a much higher risk of heart attack.

If your doctor has diagnosed you with sleep apnea—and that can happen only after a thorough examination of your sleeping habits—you probably have been made aware of the risks. But here are some remedies you should also note.

Lighten your load. It's no wonder that nearly *all* of those with sleep apnea are overweight. "Often, losing weight *alone* is enough to solve the problem," says Dr. Hauri. That's because fat deposits in the obese—particularly men—are at the base of the tongue. The extra fatty tissue blocks an already clogged air passage, making nighttime breathing more difficult.

Say no to nightcaps. Drinking in the evening is never a good idea for snorers, but it's particularly dangerous for those with sleep apnea. Research by Merrill Mitler, Ph.D., director of research for the Division of Chest, Critical Care and Sleep Medicine at the Scripps Clinic Sleep Disorders Center in San Diego, found that drinking can *double* your episodes of sleep apnea compared with going to bed sober.

"You should limit alcohol for at least six hours before going to sleep," says Bernard DeBerry, M.D., a Laguna Hills, California, surgeon who specializes in procedures related to snoring and sleep apnea and who is clinical associate professor of surgery in the Head and Neck Division at the University of California, Irvine, College of Medicine. "Alcohol is a central nervous system depressant, and as such, it decreases control of muscles in your upper airway." The more "relaxed" those muscles are, the more snoring—and the greater chance that the person with sleep apnea will stop breathing.

Get off your back. If you have sleep apnea, that's the worst position to sleep in. Once again, the culprit is gravity, says Quentin Regestein, M.D., director of the Sleep Clinic at Boston's Brigham and Women's Hospital. Sleeping on your side or your stomach will help you breathe by preventing your tongue from falling back into your throat. To make sure you stay off your back, pin a sock with a tennis ball inside the back of your pajamas, he suggests. When you try to roll over in your sleep—Bump!—the ball will wake you up.

Wear a mask. A relatively new technique called continuous positive airway pressure has revolutionized the treatment of sleep apnea, Dr. Regestein says. While people sleep, a machine pumps air into a face mask they don before going to bed. The increased air pressure "works wonderfully to prevent apneas," he says.

TINNITUS

For most people, the rhythmic sound of ocean waves caressing the shore is as soothing as a mother's lullaby. But if that splish-splash-hiss-crash is *inside* your ears, it's a different story. Tinnitus, or "ringing in the ears," is the name of *that* lullaby. And it's anything but soothing!

Tinnitus is not a disease, and it doesn't cause hearing disorders. Instead, it's any kind of swishing, hissing, whirring, ringing, whistling, buzzing or chirping that goes on inside your head.

The causes? Tinnitus can be a sign of hearing loss, or it can result from head injuries, ear infections or diseases that range from the common cold to diabetes. People who work with noisy equipment, such as power tools, can also get it. Or tinnitus may be initiated by a single loud noise, such as a gunshot or an explosion.

Sometimes tinnitus is only temporary. If you have a ringing in your ears for only a few days (perhaps after listening to loud music), take it as a warning sign. Tone down your listening habits or tinnitus may become permanent.

Even when tinnitus moves in to stay, there are still things you can do about it. The first move is a medical checkup. After that, here are some ways to make it easier to live with.

Tone down sound around you. "*Never* expose your ears to loud sounds, because they simply make tinnitus worse," says Jack Vernon, Ph.D., professor of otolaryngology at Oregon Health Sciences University and director of the Oregon Hearing Research Center, both in Portland. "If you have to raise your voice to be heard, then the sound around you is too loud. That includes vacuum cleaners, dishwashers, lawn mowers and so forth."

So wear earplugs whenever noise abounds. Pharmacies carry foam, rubber and moldable wax plugs as well as headphones you wear like earmuffs.

Try a little night static. Some people don't notice their tinnitus in the daytime, but as soon as the lights go out, they're up to their inner ears in bells and buzzers. "For those folks, I recommend detuning an FM radio to static *between* stations," says Dr. Vernon. If you keep the radio near the bed, just loud enough to be audible, the static near your head will mask the sounds *in* your head and let you fall asleep. Other sounds that might be the key to dreamland: a fan running all night or a bit of soft music.

Play that shower! In the "mask that sound" department: "Some people can't hear their tinnitus when they take showers," says Dr. Vernon. Of course, you can't stay in the shower all day, but you can carry shower sounds around with you. Dr. Vernon suggests making a long-playing tape of a running shower. When the tinnitus gets bad, listen to the tape through headphones, he recommends. (The idea is to find a band of tones that includes your tinnitus tone but is more acceptable to listen to.)

Breathe deeply to dismiss distress. "Reducing stress often reduces tinnitus," says Robert E. Brummett, Ph.D., a pharmacologist at the Oregon Hearing Research Center in Portland. Deep, slow breathing is one safe way to ease tension any time you feel it creeping up on you, according to Dr. Vernon. But he cautions that this may not be enough. See a counselor if you're having difficulty dealing with stress in your life and your tinnitus is becoming worse because of it.

Skip the smokes and drinks. "Restrict the nicotine, alcohol, tonic water and caffeine you consume," Dr. Brummett says. If you find that it helps to cut out one or all of these, consider a permanent vacation from the noise provoker.

Don't take aspirin. People with tinnitus who take aspirin daily (for arthritis, for example) should try a different anti-inflammatory drug if possible, says Dr. Brummett. Aspirin can cause or worsen tinnitus. Some of the other anti-inflammatory drugs can also cause or worsen tinnitus, but not in everyone. By working with your doctor, you can try some of the alternative drugs until you find one that you can tolerate.

Give yourself a dose of distraction. "Getting distracted from tinnitus surely will help," says Dr. Vernon. "Focus on some outside things: Help other people. Join some volunteer groups. Don't retire!" he suggests. "People with tinnitus need to enrich rather than restrict their lives."

Try a hearing aid. It's been known for some time that a hearing aid can reduce tinnitus noise—studies show up to two-thirds of people who've tried them reported reduction or total elimination of tinnitus. Why? No one knows for sure, but it may be that amplified outside noise masks the inner noise. Or at least for people whose hearing is normal or near normal, the noise produced by the hearing aid's electronic circuitry may cancel out the tinnitus.

Give your tinnitus some feedback. Biofeedback training can teach you to relax to the point that your tinnitus may become more tolerable. Studies show that the majority of tinnitus sufferers benefit from biofeedback; they sleep better and need fewer tranquilizers and antidepressants.

TRIGLYCERIDE CONTROL

What with smoking and cholesterol and blood pressure and stress and HDL and LDL and obesity and genes, figuring out your heart disease risk is pretty complicated—so why not toss another risk factor like triglycerides into the picture?

Think of triglycerides as too much of a good thing. Along with cholesterol, triglycerides are the major source of fat circulating in the blood. And just as cholesterol is needed to protect nerves and build strong cells and hormones, triglycerides are necessary for producing your body's energy. But that doesn't mean they're always beneficial. On the contrary, when triglycerides get too high, you increase your risk of heart disease, because there's too much fat in your blood.

Among older women participating in the Framingham Heart Study in Massachusetts, those who had heart disease also tended to have high triglycerides. But these same women also tended to be dangerously overweight, making it hard to pin the rap for heart disease on high triclygerides alone, says Virgil Brown, M.D., an official of the American Heart Association.

So do you have to be concerned about your triglycerides or not? A bit—if only because high triglycerides rarely come alone. "High triglycerides are often associated with obesity and several other important risk factors, such as a high-fat diet and sedentary lifestyle," says Dr. Brown.

In general, you need to get the level down if your triglycerides are over 500 milligrams per deciliter (mg/dl). But any level between 250 and 500 mg/dl is considered borderline, and most doctors think it's best to keep levels below 150. Here's how.

Gobble up garlic. Studies show that eating as little as one clove a day can lower triglyceride production. And the more you eat, the better the effect. "Studies on lab animals show that a diet made of 2 percent garlic—the equivalent of three to five cloves per day for the average American—can reduce triglycerides 25 to 30 percent," says Yu-Yan Yeh, Ph.D., associate professor of nutrition at Pennsylvania State University in University Park and a leading researcher on the healing properties of garlic. "What garlic does is lower production of triglycerides as well as reduce their release from the liver into the blood." (It can also reduce cholesterol as much as 15 percent, he notes.)

Fresh or powdered? It doesn't even matter. *Any* garlic is good garlic.

Feed on fish. Besides garlic, a diet rich in certain fish has been shown to lower triglyceride levels in some people. "We did a fish oil study and found that even people with low or below-normal trigylcerides saw a reduction after eating a lot of fish oil, which is rich in omega-3 fatty acids," says Beverly Clevidence, Ph.D., research nutritionist at the U.S. Department of Agriculture Human Nutrition Research Center's Lipid Lab in Beltsville, Maryland.

For best results, however, you need to consume about 15 grams of fish oil a day—the amount in eight ounces of salmon, mackerel or herring, the best sources of omega-3s.

Make your carbs complex. There's no question that simple carbohydrates such as candy, sugars and other sweets boost triglycerides. Besides, they provide "empty" calories that are high in fat but low in nutrition.

For effective dieting and triglyceride control, Dr. Clevidence suggests replacing fats with complex carbohydrates: "You get a lot of vitamins and nutrients for the calories." That means eating a lot of grains and pasta dishes as well as plenty of fresh fruits and vegetables.

Go easy on alcohol. Even in small amounts, booze has a damaging effect. "That's because the liver often converts alcohol into blood fats," says Dr. Clevidence. "Something like one in three people who have high triglycerides can lower them by staying away from alcohol."

WHEN NOTHING BUT RICE IS NICE

E ven its developer called it disagreeable medicine. In fact, said Walter Kempner, M.D., there's only one excuse for ever using it. "It helps."

The year was 1944, and the disagreeable medicine Dr. Kempner was speaking of was the rice diet he'd just discovered. Some of his most critically ill patients had apparently been cured by eating a diet of almost nothing but rice and fruit.

Forms of that diet are still in use today, and some call it a forerunner of the healthy-for-your-heart Pritikin Diet, among others. In some places, the rice/fruit diet is still being recommended for its ability to reduce fats from the blood and lower body weight.

"We use the rice/fruit diet in people with really high triglyceride levels to clear them out," says Sonja Connor, M.S., R.D. "It also helps them with weight loss, because it's practically fat-free.

"People don't have much of a tolerance for it," she adds.

Yet some people can apparently tolerate a steady diet of rice and fruit long enough to have an effect. "We had a patient recently who went from blood triglyceride levels of 1,000 mg/dl down to 117 mg/dl in a couple of months," says Connor. "And she went out and did this herself using that diet—we didn't have to supervise her at all." But, Connor notes, "she wasn't the typical patient."

A diet this extreme should never be attempted without the approval of your doctor, however. And most doctors are not crazy about recommending it.

How long must you subsist on rice and fruit to see results? "Not long at all," Connor says. "You start getting results on this diet right away—two or three days. If we can motivate people to get rid of all fats from their diets on a short-term basis," she explains, "we could help eradicate the problem and they could start adding some fats back in."

Lose weight—even if you don't need to. Although it's well established that overweight people are usually at greatest risk of high triglycerides, "some normal-weight people can lower their triglycerides by losing weight—even if it's just a few pounds," says Dr. Clevidence. "We're not exactly sure why it occurs, but for some people, it does."

If you're overweight, dieting is probably the best way to reduce triglycerides. Along with a regular exercise program—one hour of exercise at least three times a week—it's best to limit total dietary fat intake to about 20 percent of total daily calories. But even if fat intake is around 30 percent, you'll probably see some benefits, says Robert DiBianco, M.D., associate clinical professor of medicine at Georgetown University in Washington, D.C., and director of the Cardiac Risk Factor Reduction Program and cardiology research at Washington Adventist Hospital in Takoma Park, Maryland.

Don't light up. Although often overlooked, smoking is one of the biggest contributors to excessive blood fats. It does damage indirectly by reducing HDL cholesterol, which helps take triglycerides from the blood back into the liver for excretion. "With fewer HDLs, there are more of the undesirable blood fats, including higher levels of triglycerides," says Dr. Clevidence.

ULCERS

If ever an ailment was designed to test our patience, it's this one. Ulcers are the ultimate hang-around, come-and-go, now-you-feel-it-now-you-don't kind of problem.

If you could peek inside your stomach, however, you'd see the problem at once. Ulcers are raw, craterlike spots in the stomach or just beyond the stomach in the part of the intestine called the duodenum.

They occur when, for one reason or another, the cells normally lining the stomach or intestine no longer provide protection against the caustic effects of stomach acid. The stomach literally digests itself.

Only a doctor can tell you for sure whether you have ulcers. And even the best of doctors can't tell you exactly when you're going to have a flare-up.

But here are some self-care steps to take when you feel your ulcers going into overdrive, along with some tips that could help your ulcers heal faster.

Multiply and divide your meals. Food neutralizes the stomach acid that causes ulcers, so you may be able to reduce ulcer pain by eating more frequently. Some people have less ulcer upset if they eat six small meals a day instead of three full-size meals, according to Thomas Brasitus, M.D., professor of medicine and director of gastroenterology at the University of Chicago Pritzker School of Medicine.

Banish the food culprits. Doctors used to supply a hit list of foods to strike from the diet, including a lot of yummy fare. No longer. Now it's up to you to decide.

"The foods that bother people seem to vary with each individual," says David Earnest, M.D., professor of medicine at the University of Arizona College of Medicine Health Sciences Center in Tucson and chairman of the Clinical Practice Section for the American Gastroenterological Association.

Those foods *might* be the classic arsonists such as pepperoni pizza and very hot chili. "Obviously, spicy foods may bother some people," says Dr. Earnest. But foods that sound soothing, such as milk, ice cream or chicken soup, could be part of the problem. So play watchdog with your diet, and drop the symptom aggravators from your menu.

Use over-the-counter antacids. These drugs can heal an ulcer, at least temporarily, according to Naurang Agrawal, M.D., staff gastroenterologist at the Ochsner Clinic in New Orleans. To help ease ulcer discomfort, try the following schedule: Take two tablespoons of antacid one hour after a meal, three hours after a meal, at bedtime and whenever you have pain.

Antacids are safe, although high doses may cause diarrhea or constipation, according to Dr. Agrawal.

Try stress relief. "Classic studies have presented strong evidence of a stress component in ulcer development," according to Steven Fahrion, Ph.D., clinical psychologist and director of the Center for Applied Psychophysiology at the Menninger Clinic in Topeka, Kansas.

Not all researchers agree. But studies suggest that stress *increases* stomach acid production and *decreases* blood flow. And if there's anything an ulcer-prone stomach doesn't need, it's more acid.

Many stress relief techniques are recommended by doctors, including deep breathing, moderate physical exercise and mind relaxation techniques such as meditation, yoga, visualization or listening to relaxation tapes.

For ulcer sufferers, Dr. Fahrion recommends a stomach-warming technique. Spend some time every day in a quiet, relaxed state and try to visualize warmth, increased blood flow and decreased acid secretion in the stomach area. This technique can "relax" blood vessels, allowing greater blood flow to the stomach area.

Puff no more. Smokers are twice as likely to get ulcers as nonsmokers. And when they do get them, studies show, the ulcers take longer to heal and will be more than three times as likely to recur.

What's the best way to quit smoking? "I offer my patients nicotine gum, but that's not enough," according to Howard Mertz, M.D., associate director of the University of California, Los Angeles, Center for Functional Bowel Disorders and Abdominal Pain. "Those who simply go cold turkey seem to be the most successful."

Avoid aspirin and ibuprofen. Over-the-counter pain relievers that fall under the category of nonsteroidal anti-inflammatory drugs (NSAIDs) should be off-limits for anyone who has ulcers, according to Dr. Agrawal.

"Even when they're taken with food or taken in 'buffered' form, they can cause the stomach lining to deteriorate to the point where ulcers form," he says.

If you need to use a pain reliever, try acetaminophen (Tylenol) instead: It's not an NSAID.

Note: Some prescription drugs, including many of those used to treat arthritis, are also ulcer-aggravating NSAIDs. But check with your doctor before you stop taking any prescribed medication.

INDEX

Note: Underscored page references indicate boxed text.

A

Acetaminophen, 17, 24, 64
Acidic food, 58, 100
Adult-onset diabetes, 41
Advil. *See* Ibuprofen
Aerobic exercise, in controlling
  arthritis, 12-13
  diverticulosis, 43
  emphysema, 51
  high blood pressure, 80
Air conditioning, hay fever relief
  and, 69-70
Air temperature changes, skin
  reactions and, 47
Air travel, phlebitis and, 95
Alcohol, effects on
  arrhythmias, 74
  cataracts, 24
  diabetes, 40
  diverticulosis, 43
  gout, 63-64
  intermittent claudication, 87
  prostate problems, 99
  psoriasis, 103
  Raynaud's syndrome, 109-10
  sleep apnea, 114-15
  tinnitus, 117
  triglyceride levels, 120
Allergies
  asthma and, 16
  chronic fatigue syndrome and,
    31
  food, 1, 2-3, 70
  hay fever, 1, 68-69
  insect, 1-2
  nickel, 47
  prostate problems and, 100

All-or-none thinking, avoiding, 35
American Academy of Allergy and
  Immunology, 1
American Diabetes Association, 39
American Lung Association, 52
Analgesics. *See specific types*
Anger, high blood pressure and, 80
Angina, 4-6
Antacids, 16-17, 57, 124
Antidiarrheal medicines, 84-85, 92
Antihistamines, 68-69, 100
Anti-inflammatory drugs, 11, 117.
  See also specific types
Antioxidants, 5. *See also specific
  types*
Antiperspirants, 45
Antiscratching therapy, 46
Anxiety, 7, 8, 9-10
Apple cider, 104
Arrhythmias, 73-76
Arthritis
  asthma problems and, 17
  carpal tunnel syndrome vs., 21
  controlling
    aerobic exercise, 12-13
    aspirin, 15
    copper bracelets, 13
    dancing, 14-15
    dehumidifier, 12
    exercise, 13-14, 14-15
    fish, 11
    food, 14
    heat packs, 15
    ibuprofen, 15
    ice packs, 15
    relaxation techniques, 14
    vegetables, 11

water exercise, 13-14
weight loss, 14
Zostrix, 12
incidence of, 11
inflammatory (rheumatoid
arthritis), 11, 83
noninflammatory
(osteoarthritis), 11, 12, 21
Aspirin
in controlling
angina, 5
arthritis, 15
blood clots, 5
heart attack, 5
intermittent claudication, 86-
87
phlebitis, 94
pneumonia, 98
effects on
gout, 64
gums, 66
tinnitus, 117
ulcers, 125
enteric-coated, 57
side effects of, 5
Astemizole, 100
Asthma, 16-18, 17
Audiotapes, relaxation, 10
Azulfidine, 82-83

B
Baby lotions, 47
Bag Balm, 104
Baking soda, 45, 67, 104
Bathing, 44, 46, 103-4
Beano, 90
Beans, 28
Beer, 64, 87. *See also* Alcohol
Bees, allergies to, 1-2
Benign prostatic hyperplasia
(BPH), 99
Benzocaine, 67

Beta-carotene, 23, 50
Biofeedback, 110, 118
Blood clots, 5, 87, 94
Blood fat, 78, 119-20, 121, 122
Blood pressure
glaucoma and, 60
gout and, 62-63
high, 77-80, 79
Blood sugar, 24, 41
Body building, 51
Body fat. *See* Overweight
BPH (benign prostatic
hyperplasia), 99
Breakfast, eating, 26, 39
Breathing
arrhythmia control and, 75
controlled, 9
from diaphragm, 50
exercises, 50-51
sleep apnea and, 114
weight training and, 51
Brushing teeth, 65

C
Caffeine, effects on
arrhythmias, 74
asthma, 18
cholesterol, 27
diverticulosis, 43
gastritis, 58
irritable bowel syndrome, 92
prostate problems, 99
Raynaud's syndrome, 109
Calcium, 78-79
Calming techniques.
See Relaxation techniques
Capsaicin, 12
Carbohydrates, 120
Carbon monoxide, angina and, 6
Cardiac arrhythmias, 73-76
Carmol 10, 46
Carmol 20, 46

Carpal tunnel, 19
Carpal tunnel syndrome, 19-22, 21
Carrots, 28-29
Cataracts, 23-24
Catastrophic thinking, avoiding, 7, 9
Celery, high blood pressure reduction and, 77
CFS (chronic fatigue syndrome), 30-32
Chills, 106-10
Chlorine, skin reactions and, 48
Cholesterol
  angina and, 4
  caffeine's effects on, 27
  controlling
    beans, 28
    breakfast, 26
    carrots, 28-29
    diet, 25-29
    fiber, 28, 39-40
    garlic, 27, 78
    grapefruit, 27
    grapes, 27
    low-fat diet, 29
    olive oil, 29
    snacking, 26-27
    vitamin C, 26
    vitamin E, 25-26
  dietary, 28
  excess, 25, 55
  gallstones and, 25, 55
  high-density lipoprotein and, 25, 26, 28, 29, 86, 122
  low-density lipoprotein and, 25, 26, 27, 28, 29
  serum, 28
  understanding, 28
Christmas trees, skin reactions to live, 47
Chromium, 40

Chronic fatigue syndrome (CFS), 30-32
Chronic glaucoma, 54
Cigarettes. See Smoking
Cilia, 97
Cimetidine, 58, 75
Cinnamon, 40-41
Circulation problems
  phlebitis, 93-95, 94
  Raynaud's syndrome, 106-10
Citrucel, 92
Cleansers, skin, 44
Clothing
  drying, 70
  emphysema and, 52
  Gore-Tex, 108
  hats, 23, 118
  hay fever and, 70
  mittens, 109
  Raynaud's syndrome and, 107-9
Coal tar preparations, 104
Coffee, 18, 27. See also Caffeine
Cold medicines, 100
Cold temperatures, 6, 106-7
Colitis, ulcerative, 81, 82, 83
Colon, 42, 81, 89
Competition, arrhythmias and, 74
Contac, 60
Continuous positive airway pressure, 115
Contraceptives, oral, 94-95
Control, need for, 10
Copper bracelets, arthritis control and, 13
Cortisone, 60
Cosmetics, skin reactions and, 48
Coughing, 97
Counseling, 32
Crohn's and Colitis Foundation of America, 85
Crohn's disease, 81-82, 83
Curry, diabetes control and, 40-41

D

Dairy products, 91
Dancing, 14-15
Decaffeinated coffee, 27
Decongestants, 75, 100
Deep-vein thrombophlebitis, 95
Dehumidifier, arthritis control
    and, 12
Dental problems, 65-67
Deodorants, skin reactions and, 45
Depression, 33-36
Dermatitis, 44-46, 47, 48
Diabetes
    adult-onset, 41
    alcohol's effects on, 40
    cataracts and, 24
    controlling
        breakfast, 39
        cinnamon, 40-41
        exercise, 38
        fiber, 39-40
        low-fat diet, 38-39
        muscle building, 38
        snacking, 39
        tumeric, 40-41
        weight loss, 37-38
        weight training, 38
    hypoglycemia and, 41
    insulin-dependent, 37
    non-insulin-dependent, 37
    overweight and, 37
    Type I, 37
    Type II, 37
Dial soap, 45
Diaphragm, 49, 50
Diarrhea, 82, 84, 85
Diet. *See also* Low-fat diet
    in controlling
    fad, avoiding, 38
    no-fat, 54
    rice, 121
    ulcers and, 123

vegetarian, 4, 11
Dietary fat, 4, 11, 38, 54.
    See also Cholesterol
Digestive problems
    colitis, 81, 82, 83
    Crohn's disease, 81-82, 83
    diverticulitis, 42
    diverticulosis, 42-43
    gallstones, 25, 53-54
    gastritis, 56-58
    inflammatory bowel disease, 81-
        85
    irritable bowel syndrome, 89-
        92, 90
    ulcers, 58, 122-25
Dining out, hearing loss and, 71-
    72
Dipentum, 83
Diverticulitis, 42
Diverticulosis, 42-43
Drug-related depression, 36
Drugs. *See* Medications; *specific
    types*
Dryer sheets, skin reactions and, 48
Drying clothes, hay fever and, 70
Duodenum, 123

E

Ear plugs, 72, 116
Ear problems
    hearing loss, 71-72
    tinnitus, 116-18
Ear protectors, 72, 116
Ectopic atrial heartbeat, 73
Eczema, 44-46, 47, 48
Ejaculation, 100-101
Electric razor, psoriasis and, 105
Electric tools, avoiding, 20
Emollients, 46
Emotional problems
    anxiety, 7, 8, 9-10
    depression, 33-36

Emotional problems *(continued)*
  seasonal affective disorder, 111,
    112, 113
Emphysema, 16, 49-52
Ephedrine, 75
Eucerin cream, 102
Exercise. *See also* Aerobic exercise
  body building, 51
  carbon monoxide inhalation
    during outdoor, 6
  in cold temperatures, 6
  in controlling
    anxiety, 10
    arthritis, 13-14, 14-15
    carpal tunnel syndrome, 19-
      20
    chronic fatigue syndrome,
      30-31
    depression, 33
    diabetes, 38
    glaucoma, 60
    intermittent claudication, 87-
      88
    osteoarthritis, 12
    Raynaud's syndrome, 107
  dancing, 14-15
  hypoglycemia and, 41
  isometric, 80
  muscle building, 38
  in preventing
    angina, 5
    arrhythmias, 73-74
  running, 43
  walking, 87-88, 113
  water, 13-14, 48
  weight training, 38, 51
  yoga, 113
Expectorants, 98
Eyedrops, 59-60
Eye exam, 61
Eye problems
  cataracts, 23-24

glaucoma, 59-61, 61

F

Fabric softener, skin reactions and,
  48
Fad diet, avoiding, 38
Fat, body. *See* Overweight
Fat, dietary, 4, 11, 38, 54. *See also*
  Cholesterol
Fears, 8. *See also* Anxiety
Fever, 66
Fiber
  in controlling
    cholesterol, 28, 39-40
    diabetes, 39-40
    diverticulosis, 42
    inflammatory bowel disease,
      84
    irritable bowel syndrome, 91
  gas and, 42
  water-soluble, 40
Fingernail products, skin reactions
  and, 47
Fish
  asthma prevention and, 17-18
  in controlling
    arrhythmias, 76
    arthritis, 11
    gallstones, 55
    intermittent claudication, 86
    psoriasis, 105
    triglyceride levels, 120
Fish oil, 55, 120
5-ASA, 83
Flatulence, 42, 84, 90
Fluid intake, 91, 98. *See also*
  specific types
Food. *See also* Diet; Snacking,
  specific types
  acidic, 58, 100
  allergies, 1, 2-3, 70
  arthritis and, 14

gas-producing, 84
gout-causing, 63
insect allergies and, 2
iron-rich, 107
junk, 31
psoriasis and, 105
spicy, 100
ulcers and, 123
Food diary, 3
Foot powder, 109
Framingham Heart Study, 119
Fructose, 90
Fruit juices, 54, 90-91. *See also*
    Orange juice
Fruits, 50. *See also specific types*

G
Gallbladder, 53
Gallstones, 25, 53-54
Garlic, in controlling
    cholesterol, 27, 78
    high blood pressure, 77-78
    triglyceride levels, 119-20
Garlic pills, 27
Garments. *See* Clothing
Gas, 42, 84, 90
Gastritis, 56-58
Glaucoma, 59-61, 61
Glucose, 37, 41
Goal-setting, 9-10, 35
Gore-Tex, 108
Gout, 62-64, 63
Grapefruit, 27
Grapes, 27
Gum pain, 65-67

H
Hand-arm vibration syndrome, 20
Hats, 23, 108
Hay fever, 1, 68-69
HDL (high-density lipoprotein),
    25, 26, 28, 29, 86, 122

Hearing aids, 71, 118
Hearing loss, 71-72
Heart attack, 5, 115
Heart problems. *See also* Angina
    arrhythmias, 73-76
    heart attack, 5, 115
    triglyceride levels and, 119
Heat packs
    in controlling
        arthritis, 15
        carpal tunnel syndrome, 22
        irritable bowel syndrome, 92
        intermittent claudication and,
            88
High blood pressure, 77-80, 79
High-density lipoprotein (HDL),
    25, 26, 28, 29, 86, 122
Hismanal, 100
Home blood pressure monitor, 79
Humidifier, dermatitis/eczema
    and, 46
Humidity, controlling, 12, 46
Hydrocortisone cream, 46
Hydrogen peroxide, 67
Hypertension, 77-80, 79
Hypoglycemia, 41

I
IBD (inflammatory bowel
    disease), 81-85
IBS (irritable bowel syndrome),
    89-92, 90
Ibuprofen
    cataract prevention and, 24
    in controlling
        arthritis, 15
        asthma, 17
        gout, 64
        gum pain, 66
    ulcers and, effects on, 125
Ice packs in controlling
    arthritis, 15

Ice packs in controlling *(continued)*
  carpal tunnel syndrome, 22
  dermatitis, 44-45
  eczema, 44-45
  gum pain, 66
Immunosuppressants, 83
Immunotherapy, 2
Imodium, 85
Indigestion, 56, 57-58
Inflammatory arthritis, 11
Inflammatory bowel disease
  (IBD), 81-85
Insects, allergies to, 1-2
Insulin, 26, 37, 41
Insulin-dependent diabetes, 37
Intermittent claudication, 86-88
Iron, 107
Irritable bowel syndrome (IBS),
  89-92, 90
Isometric exercise, 80

J

Jewelry, skin reactions and, 47
Joint problems, 62-64, 63. *See also*
  Arthritis
Juicers, 90
Juices, fruit, 54, 90-91. *See also*
  Orange juice
Junk food, 31

K

Kyolic, 27

L

Lac-Hydrin Five, 46
Lactic acid, 46, 102
LactiCare, 102
Lactose intolerance, 91
Laundry detergents, 46
Laxatives, 92
LDL (low-density lipoprotein),
  25, 27, 28, 29

Leg problems
  intermittent claudication, 86-88
  phlebitis, 93-95, 94
Legumes, 28
Light box, 112
Light therapy, 111, 112, 113
Listerine, 65
Lomotil, 85
Low-density lipoprotein (LDL),
  25, 27, 28, 29
Low-fat diet in controlling
  cholesterol, 29
  chronic fatigue syndrome, 31
  diabetes, 38-39
  gallstones, 53, 54
  gastritis, 57-58
  intermittent claudication, 86
Lungs, 49. *See also* Pulmonary
  problems
Lying, high blood pressure and, 80

M

Maalox, 84
Magnesium, 31
Masking sounds, 116-17
Massage, 65, 94
Meat, red, 4, 63
Medications. *See also* Over-the-
  counter medications
  cold, 100
  effects on
    arrhythmias, 75
    depression, 36
    glaucoma, 60
    irritable bowel syndrome, 92
  inflammatory bowel disease, 82
Meditation, 9, 92
Melons, 70
Metabolic overload, 74, 84
Metamucil, 42, 92
Microwave, cataracts and, 24
Milk

in controlling
gastritis, 57
seasonal affective disorder,
113
intolerance to, 91
Milk compress, 45
Mittens, 109
Moisturel Sensitive Skin Cleanser,
44
Moisturizing skin, 48, 102-3
Mucus, 97, 98
Multivitamins, 31
Muscle building, 38

N
Nail care, 45
Nasal sprays, 69
Negative thinking, avoiding faulty,
35
Nerve problems, 19-22, 21
Nickel allergies, 47
Nicotine, 87. *See also* Smoking
Nicotine gum, 125
Nitroglycerin pill, 5, 6
No-fat diet, 54
Noninflammatory arthritis, 11,
12, 21
Non-insulin-dependent diabetes,
37
Nonsteroidal anti-inflammatory
drugs (NSAIDs)
asthma and, 17, 125
Nutrients, 18

O
Oatmeal baths, 44, 46
Obesity, 119. *See also* Overweight
Olive oil, 29, 54-55, 103
Omega-3 fatty acids, 11, 18, 76,
120
Oral contraceptives, 94-95
Orange juice, 23-24, 41

Osteoarthritis, 11, 12, 21. *See also*
Arthritis
Overeating, 74, 84
Over-the-counter medications.
See also Aspirin
antidiarrheal, 84-85, 92
coal tar, 104
expectorants, 98
fever, 66
gum pain, 66, 67
ulcer, 124
Overweight
arthritis and, 14
diabetes and, 37
gallstones and, 53-54
gout and, 62
sleep apnea and, 114
triglyceride levels and, 122

P
Pain relievers. *See specific types*
Palpitations, heart, 73-76
Parasympathetic nerves, 75
Pectin, 27, 29
Perfectionism, avoiding, 10
Personalizing, avoiding, 35
Perspiration, 107-8
Pets, 47, 79
Phlebitis, 93-95, 94
Phlegm, 97, 98
Phobias, 8. *See also* Anxiety
the Pill, 94
Plaques, 102, 105
Pneumonia, 96-98
Pollen counts, 69
Polyunsaturated fat, 11
Positive action, 34
Potassium, 78
Progressive relaxation, 9, 109
Prostate problems, 99-101
Pseudoephedrine, 75
Psoriasis, 102-5

Psyllium products, 42, 92
Pulmonary problems
asthma, 16-18, <u>17</u>
emphysema, 16, 49-52
pneumonia, 96-98
Purine, 63, 64

R

Radiation, 23-24
Raynaud's syndrome, 106-10
Reflux, stomach, 16
Relaxation techniques
audiotapes, 10
biofeedback, 110, 118
in controlling
anxiety, 9, 10
arrhythmias, 76
arthritis, 14
dermatitis, 48
eczema, 48
irritable bowel syndrome, 92
Raynaud's syndrome, 109
ulcers, 124
meditation, 9, 92
progressive relaxation, 9, 109
stomach-warming, 124
yoga, 113
Repetitive movement, 19
Respiratory infections, 101
Rheumatoid arthritis, 11, 83.
See also Arthritis
Rice diet, <u>121</u>
Ringing in the ears, 116-18
Running, 43

S

SAD (seasonal affective disorder),
111, <u>112</u>, 113
Saliva, replenishing, 66-67
Salt intake, 63, 78
Salt water, inhaling for hay fever
relief, 69

Saltwater rinse, 66
Saturated fat, 4, 54
Seasonal affective disorder (SAD),
111, <u>112</u>, 113
Seldane, 100
Self-defining questions, asking,
35-36
Self-esteem, improving, 34
Serum cholesterol, <u>28</u>
Sexual activity, 64, 100
Shampooing hair, 70
Shaving, 105
Shoes, 2, 64, 108
Simethicone, 84
Skin problems
dermatitis, 44-46, <u>47</u>, 48
eczema, 44-46, <u>47</u>, 48
psoriasis, 102-5
Skipping meals, avoiding, 38, <u>41</u>
Sleep apnea, 114-15
Sleeping
angina and, 6
asthma and, 17
carpal tunnel syndrome and, 21
chronic fatigue syndrome and,
32
depression and, 33-34
inflammatory bowel disease
and, 84
pneumonia and, 98
prostate problems and, 101
sleep apnea and, 115
Smoking
effects on
arrhythmias, 73
asthma, 16
cataracts, 24
diverticulosis, 43
emphysema, 49, 51
gastritis, 58
gum pain, 67
intermittent claudication, 87

phlebitis, 95
pneumonia, 97
Raynaud's syndrome, 109
tinnitus, 117
triglyceride levels, 122
ulcers, 124-25
quitting, 125
Snacking, in controlling
asthma, 16-17
cholesterol, 26-27
diabetes, 39
emphysema, 49-50
Snoring, 114, 115
Soap, skin reactions to, 45
Sodium intake, 63, 78
Soltriol, 113
Sorbitol, 90
Sounds, 71-72, 116-17
Spastic colon, 89-92, <u>90</u>
Speaking, high blood pressure and,
80
Spicy food, 100
Steroids, 83
Stockings, 88, 95
Stomach acid, 16-17, 57
Stomach problems. *See* Digestive
problems
Streptococcus pneumoniae, 96
Stress, effects on
arrhythmias, 74, 76
dermatitis, 48
eczema, 48
inflammatory bowel disease, 85
irritable bowel syndrome, 89, 92
prostate problems, 100
psoriasis, 105
Raynaud's syndrome, 109
tinnitus, 117
ulcers, 124
Stress diary, 89, 92
Stuffed animals, skin reactions
and, <u>47</u>

Sugar, <u>41</u>, 90-91
Sulfasalazine, 82-83
Sunglasses, cataract prevention
and, 23-24
Sunlight
artificial, 103, 111, <u>112</u>, 113
UV protection and, 23-24
Superficial phlebitis, 93
Supplements, 40
Support hose, 95
Support, social
chronic fatigue syndrome and,
32
depression and, 34
emphysema and, 52
inflammatory bowel disease
and, 85
Surgery, prostate, 99
Sweat glands, 107
Sweets, <u>41</u>, 90-91
Swimming, 13-14, 48
Sympathetic nerves, 75-76

T

Tagamet, 58, 75
Tanning booths, 103
Tea leaves, 67
Terfenadine, 100
Theophylline, 17, 18
Thrombophlebitis, 93-95, <u>94</u>
Tinnitus, 116-18
Tobacco, chewing, 67. *See also*
Smoking
Toilet paper, colored, <u>47</u>
Tomatoes, 105
Tom's of Maine Natural
Deodorant, 45
Tools, carpal tunnel syndrome
and, 20
Tooth problems. *See* Dental
problems
Trench mouth, 67

Triglycerides, 78, 119-20, <u>121</u>, 122
Turmeric, 40-41
Tylenol. *See* Acetaminophen
Type I diabetes, 37
Type II diabetes, 37

U

Ulcerative colitis, 81, 82, 83
Ulcers, 58, 122-25
Ultra Mide 25, 46
Urea, 46
Urethra, 99
Uric acid, 62, 63, 64
Urination, 64, 99, 100
Utility cart, for housework, 52
UV protection, 23-24

V

Vagal maneuver, 75-76
Vagal nerves, 75-76
Vegetable oil, 103-4
Vegetables, 11, 50. *See also specific types*
Vegetarian diet, 4, 11
Vitamin A, 5
Vitamin B$_6$, 20-21
Vitamin C
  cataract prevention and, 23
  in controlling
    angina, 5
    asthma, 18
    cholesterol, 26
    emphysema, 50
    glaucoma, 60-61
  sources of, 18, 50
Vitamin D, 113
Vitamin E
  cataract prevention and, 23
  in controlling
    angina, 5

  cholesterol, 25-26
  sources of, 23, 26
Vitamins. *See also specific types*
  in controlling
    angina, 5
    asthma, 18
    chronic fatigue syndrome, 31
  deficiencies in, B-vitamins, 20-21

W

Walking, 87-88, 113
Water exercise, 13-14, 48
Water intake
  diverticulosis and, 43
  gout and, 64
  irritable bowel syndrome and, 91
Weight loss
  in controlling
    arthritis, 14
    diabetes, 37-38
    gallstones, 53-54
    gout, 62
    triglyceride levels, 122
  emphysema and, 49-50
  gradual, 38, 54
Weight training, 38, 51
Wine, 64, 87. *See also* Alcohol
Work, 20, 52
Workouts. *See* Exercise
Wrist splint, 21

Y

Yoga, 113
Yuppie flu, 30-32

Z

Zest soap, 45
Zinc, 18, 95
Zostrix, 12